D1038397

1-
STRAND PRICE
$ 2.00

EXERCISE or DIET

Which will win the race to health?

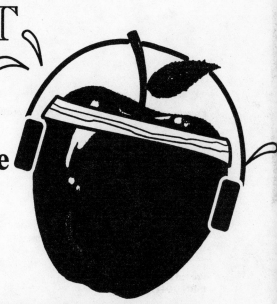

Dr. M. Ted Morter, Jr.

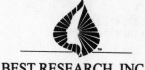

BEST RESEARCH, INC.

All rights reserved. No part of this publication may be reproduced in any form or by any means, electronic or mechanical, including photocopy, recording or any information storage and retrieval system now known or to be invented, without permission in writing from the author. For information, contact B.E.S.T. Research, Inc., 1000 West Poplar, Rogers, Arkansas 72756.

The author assumes no responsibility for inaccuracies, deficiencies, errors or omissions. It is not the intention of the author to slight or offend any individuals, groups or organizations by reference or implication. The reader should consult qualified professionals specializing in holistic health care regarding individual conditions.

Exercise or Diet: Which will win the race to health?
1997

Dr. M. Ted Morter, Jr.

Copyright © 1997, B.E.S.T. Research, Inc.

Printed in the United States
ISBN 0-944994-11-3

Morter HealthSystem
1000 West Poplar Street
Rogers, Arkansas 72756

1 800 874 1478
1 501 631 8201 (Fax)

INFORMATION FOR THE READER

The information presented in this book is a compilation of concepts and principles developed by the author over the past thirty years. These concepts and principles primarily relate to maintaining and promoting health, not to treating disease or other physical complaints. The reader is specifically cautioned against applying concepts in this book for therapeutic purposes in lieu of professional health care. The reader is urged to consult licensed health care professionals for diagnosis and treatment of health problems. This book deals with the basic concept that the body functions as a unit, that various elements of lifestyle influence physiology, and that certain physiological processes respond in a predetermined manner to specific stimuli. Consequently, certain concepts and ideas presented are intended to offer suggestions for examining facets of one's lifestyle that can impact physiology.

No guarantee or assurance is given for obtaining specific individuals to obtain specific results from the adoption of any suggestion. Regular professional health care examinations are important to early detection and treatment of all diseases. This publication deals with prevention of diseases rather than with disease treatment.

Certain persons considered experts may disagree with one or more statements in this publication. However, the author is of the opinion that such statements are based upon reliable, sound report and authority. Nothing stated in this publication shall be construed as an offer of any product for the diagnosis, cure, mitigation, or treatment of any disease.

Dr. M. Ted Morter, Jr.

Dr. Morter's latest book is a wonderful introduction on how exercise plays an important role in whole body health.

The simplistic manner of Dr. Morter's writing style combines physiological, neuromuscular, neurodevelopmental, and metaphysical concepts with exercise, and the other five essentials of whole body health in an easy to read and apply format.

After reading this book, health care providers and consumers will realize that development and rejuvenation involves more than exercising or treating separate body parts. Proper exercise, good food, clean air, sufficient rest, and a good self image are important in an individual's development. What we need to realize is that our development begins at conception, and these factors continue to affect our whole body health throughout life.

This book will give you a jump start on your road to health!

Scott Johnson
Registered Physical Therapist

BOOKS BY
M.T. MORTER, JR., M.A., D.C.

Correlative Urinalysis: The Body Knows Best. 1987, Best Research, Inc. A guide for health care professionals for evaluating, through urinalysis, the effects of excess acid ash-producing foods on physiological systems.

Chiropractic Physiology: A review of scientific principles as related to the chiropractic adjustment with emphasis on Bio Enenergetic Synchronization Technique, 1988, B.E.S.T. Research, Inc. A review for health care professionals of the impact on anatomical and physiological systems of the body of chiropractic adjustments in general, and Bioenergetic Synchronization Technique in particular.

Your Health, Your Choice: Your Complete Personal Guide to Wellness, Nutrition, and Disease Prevention, 1990, Fell Publishers, Inc. A summary of how foods we eat regularly affect how we feel, why some types of everyday foods can lead to ill-health, and ways to adjust diet shlowly to replenish vital alkalizing minerals.

The Healing Field: Restoring the Positive Energy of Health, 1991, B.E.S.T. Research, Inc. A discussion of the concept that the body is an energy being and that health is a reflection of the vitality of the energy fields in and around the body.

An Apple A Day?: Is it Enough Today?, 1997 (Rev.) B.E.S.T. Research, Inc. How the foods we eat can affect physiological responses and the acid-alkaline balance of the internal environment of the body.

Exercise or Diet: Which Will Win the Race to Health? 1997, B.E.S.T. Research, Inc. Fitness is not the same as health. Why we should exercise and when we shouldn't. Why exercise can't make you healthy but can enhance the vitality and well-being of a healthy body.

Dynamic Health: Using Your Own Beliefs, Thoughts, and Memory to Create a Healthy Body, 1997 (Rev.), B.E.S.T. Research, Inc. Health and physiology are affected by conscious thoughts and stored memories. *Dynamic Health* helps to correlate how we think with how we feel and how healthy we are.

TABLE OF CONTENTS

CHAPTER 4
MORE THAN A MEMORY

CHAPTER 5
SHAPING UP

CHAPTER 6
YOU'RE A BUNDLE OF ENERGY

CHAPTER 7
STRESSING EXERCISE

PROLOGUE

NOT JUST ANOTHER
EXERCISE BOOK

This book is about more than exercise and being fit. It's about whole-body health. It's about how exercise affects your whole body from cells to psyche. Not just your waistline, muscles, cardiorespiratory system, strength, endurance, and physique. The general attitude in our culture is that health comes from regular vigorous, sweaty exercise. This book is about why you should be healthy *before* you exercise strenuously. It relates the effects of diet and strenuous exercise on your internal environment and physiological responses. This book gives a perspective on health, exercise, and fitness that may be new to you.

Fitness has become a national obsession. But fitness is hollow glory without good health. Fitness may give you bragging rights, but good health gives you a competitive edge for success and satisfaction in life.

So, just what is good health?

Is it nothing more than being disease-free, pain-free, symptom-free, at least moderately energetic, and reasonably flexible? The World Health Organization sees health as "a state of complete physical, mental, or social well-being and not merely the absence of disease or infirmity."[1] However, as we shall see, all of the clues we give as evidence of health are really symptoms, or reflections, of health — not health itself. Good health is a "core issue" for your body. Health — for good or ill — is a reflection of the condition of your internal environment.

> WELLNESS PRINCIPLE: Health from the inside is
> reflected on the outside.

For our purposes, we'll define health as a process rather than a state of being. Health is dynamic — ever changing. Health is the ability of the body's integrated biological, chemical, and electrical systems to respond to internal and external stimuli and return to internal homeostasis without being continuously dependent on physiological backup systems. In other words, health is the process of the body meeting stimulation challenges from the inside and outside, recovering from them, and doing all of this without constantly calling on emergency reserves to handle day-to-day functions.

Exercise is one element of living that affects your health. However, we have a paradox here. Your body needs exercise to *be* healthy. But exercise can't *make* you healthy. Exercise can enhance health if your body isn't overburdened just trying to survive. A regular exercise program can help you to look better, be more energetic, more flexible, stronger, and more upbeat. Yet, even if you exercise strenuously and regularly — work out, run or walk mega-miles, play tennis or golf — you may not be healthy. Your body may be working overtime to handle the health-inhibiting effects of improper diet, polluted air, restless sleep, or persistent emotional upheaval.

Every day you make health-promoting or health-inhibiting choices in six essential areas of life — what you eat and drink, how you exercise, rest, and breathe, and what you think. You have conscious control over your decisions in each of these six areas. You decide consciously what you will eat and drink. You consciously choose how and when you will exercise and rest.

You consciously control where you live and work, which determines the quality of the air you breathe. And, you have conscious control over the attitudes and thoughts that run through (or get stuck in) your mind.

The effects of choices you make in each of these six essentials are stresses to your body. Your body must respond to the effects of your choices day after day, year after year. When your essential choices help your body to function easily and smoothly, you reap the benefits we call "health." If your conscious choices keep your body working overtime to survive, systems and organs will eventually become exhausted. There goes "health." Systems and organs can be overworked and become exhausted in the same way muscles can. When systems and organs become exhausted, like muscles, they can't function efficiently. Internal exhaustion leads to ill-health.

This book is to help you understand how exercise fits into your grand scheme of promoting health. Although we focus on exercise, rest, and breathing, all of the six essentials are so interwoven that we also touch briefly on the other three. Exercise is just one element of a healthy life. This book is to help you understand why you should pursue health first, then go after fitness. And, it's to help you get a handle on making appropriate choices in the six essentials to be the healthiest you can be. We're talking here about "healthness," not "fitness." Even those who are not top-notch-healthy can benefit from exercise appropriate to their particular level of health.

WELLNESS PRINCIPLE: Your exercise program
                      should depend on your
                      body's level of health.

The big concept is: Everything you do affects some function of your body. And, in your body, everything affects everything else. Exercise affects more than just muscles. Exercise affects your whole body.

You are more than muscles, bones, organs, and nervous systems wrapped up in your personal skin. You are an integrated being. When you are healthy, you are healthy all over. When you are sick, you are sick all over.

When you have a headache, you may feel as though you are all head. However, your whole body is involved in that headache. There's much more to your body's activity level than meets the eye — or than you can feel.

When you exercise, rest, or breathe, your whole body responds. Heart rate speeds or slows; blood pressure goes up or down; oxygen delivery to the blood stream increases or decreases; muscles contract or relax; alertness heightens or falls; energy production accelerates or subsides. Literally thousands of internal physiological responses are excited or suppressed. You live in a body that functions through a finely-tuned, well-orchestrated, integrated system of chemical and electrical responses.

WELLNESS PRINCIPLE: The sole purpose of internal
                      activity is survival.

Depending on how hard your body is working just to survive, exercise can promote health or endanger life.

Exercise temporarily adds acid to the "atmosphere" of your internal environment. If your internal environment is "toxic" from excess acid when you begin to exercise, your body may not be able to withstand the additional stress. We'll see what that means and how you can tell if you need to "clean up your internal environment" before you can exercise *safely*. Those people who need to "clean up their internal environment" should limit their exercise program to walking. Those whose internal environments are in reasonably good shape may need to change their diets, and perhaps their attitudes, as they continue to exercise strenuously. No exercise program is a one-size-fits-all.

Keep in mind as you read this book that the material presented here is not a substitute for competent medical care. It is intended to give you an overview of how exercise, rest, and breathing can affect your body. This book is not a do-it-yourself manual for self-diagnosis or treatment. It is designed to give you a view of parts of your lifestyle that could affect your health either adversely or positively.

Exercise is only one of the six essentials. In these pages, we'll look at some indicators that offer clues as to whether or not you are really healthy enough to exercise. And, of course, we'll outline a few basic exercises that are appropriate for the "fit" and "unfit" alike.

We'll begin with a look at why fitness doesn't equal health. Then we'll move on to a summary of the six essentials, followed by an investigation of what you're doing to your body when you bend, stretch, run, jump, swim, or just sit there. In short, we'll give you some clues that can indicate if you are healthy enough to exercise strenuously.

Exercise not only helps your body maintain flexibility, strength, and endurance, it can be fun. When you exercise within the health range of your body, you feel better, are more alert, think better, and generally enjoy life more. As long as you're here on this earth, you may as well be the best you can be. And the best thing about "being the best you can be" is that it is a goal that you can continually stretch. As John Ruskin writes: "The highest reward for man's toil is not what he gets for it but what he becomes by it."

Now, let's see how exercise and fitness fit into your healthness.

CHAPTER 1

THE FITNESS CRAZE

A FLURRY OF FITNESS

Fitness has become a national icon. It ranks right up there with mother, apple pie, baseball, fame, and fortune. But to be fit, you need to exercise. If most of your exercise comes from brisk walks from easy chair to refrigerator topped off by vigorous construction of a Dagwood sandwich, all timed precisely to fit into TV commercial breaks, you probably aren't as fit as you could be.

Despite all the hoopla about fitness — fitness books, magazine articles, videos, ads for exercise equipment — all too many of us fall short of being fit. Maybe we can blame our current fitness crisis on Henry Ford and Eli Olds. Thanks to them, we don't walk much any more. We don't use pedal power for daily trips to the grocery store. And, we even drive to fitness centers so we can exercise.

Just what does it mean to "be fit"?

Fitness is more than being slim, trim, and muscular. It's a physiological state that is generally judged by how well a body functions in four categories.

1. Cardiorespiratory endurance: how well the heart and blood vessels can deliver oxygen to the cells.
2. Muscular fitness: strength and endurance.

3. Flexibility: joints that move freely through their full range of motion without discomfort or pain.
4. Body composition: the amount of muscle, bone, and fat.

So, does that mean that if you score well in those four categories you are healthy?

Not necessarily. It means you are "fit." You can be "fit" without being "healthy."

We tend to think of "fitness" as being the yardstick for "health." "Fit" certainly looks healthy — leaning toward lean, agile, sculptured muscles, and strength. Yet, if being fit means being healthy, why do we so often read that a top-notch, fit, well-conditioned young athlete has dropped dead or had a heart attack? The sudden death of Russian ice skater, Sergei Grinkov, is a tragic, well-publicized example of the paradox of fitness.

Grinkov was a 28 years-old gold medal Olympic athlete trained to the hilt. Throughout his routines, he not only skated, but he picked up his partner, lifted her over his head, put her down gracefully, and made it look easy. To maintain the rigorous training schedule necessary for a skater to reach world-class level, his cardiovascular endurance must have been excellent, his muscular fitness superb, his flexibility outstanding, and his body composition at least close to ideal. But was he healthy? Apparently not, or he would be skimming over the ice today.

And basketball player Reggie Lewis wasn't exercising strenuously when he collapsed and died. He was just shooting the ball. Certainly Lewis would have been considered among the fittest of the fit.

WELLNESS PRINCIPLE: Fitness doesn't guarantee
health.

No doubt about it, fitness is desirable. Being fit can make your life more pleasant. You have a spring in your step; you can do more, and do it longer; you look good; you don't tire as easily as your "unfit" colleagues; you can make the most of more opportunities. But fitness doesn't guarantee a disease-free, pain-free long life. Nothing can guarantee that. However, being as healthy as you can be is a giant step in the right direction.

Your level of fitness doesn't necessarily determine your level of health. Exercising regularly won't make you healthy. However, when you are healthy, a consistent, sensible exercise program can help to maintain or restore fitness and enhance your feeling of well-being, your attitudes, and your life. Exercise can help you have a more pleasant and productive life, but it can't make you — or keep you — healthy. Health is a function of your internal environment. Fitness is a function of exercise.

Does that mean you don't need to be fit to be healthy?

It means that your health can't be measured by how well you move, how far you can run, how many sets of tennis you can play, how much weight you can lift, or how slim and trim you are. That's fitness. This book is about *health*. It isn't a "fitness" manual — there are plenty of those around. The purpose here is to help you understand that exercise is just one component of a healthy lifestyle. Exercise isn't the be-all, end-all of health.

WELLNESS PRINCIPLE: You can't exercise your
                                          way to health.

Your health depends on two criteria: (1) the condition of your internal environment, and (2) how, or how long, your body must adapt to handle long-term stress.

The condition of your internal environment depends on the choices you make in what you eat, drink, and breathe, how you exercise and rest, and how and what you think. Your long-term health depends on how long you consistently make appropriate or inappropriate choices. Appropriate choices allow your body to handle day-to-day stresses, then return to non-stress functioning. Inappropriate choices inflict non-stop physiological stress.

No matter what stresses your body is subjected to, it will

handle them as best it can. But it doesn't handle them to make you comfortable or healthy, happy and secure. The only purpose of anything and everything your body does is survival!

SURVIVAL IS THE NAME OF THE GAME
Health is a process. It is the process of internal responses your body makes constantly to a flood of internal and external stimuli. And every internal response your body makes is for one purpose only — survival!

> WELLNESS PRINCIPLE: The sole purpose of every internal response is survival.

Through the ages, exercise has played a role in survival. Not necessarily the kind of exercise we generally think of — aerobics, weight lifting, tennis, swimming, and the like. It's more basic than that. Exercise is movement. We were designed to move. It's a survival and defense mechanism. We must move to escape danger. And we must move to find food. One of our biggest survival needs is a constant supply of food. But we can't wait for food to come to us — we have to go get it. Our distant ancestors needed keen eye sight, physical agility, strength, and stamina to find food to eat. No supermarkets. No golden arches. No microwave meals. The ability to move was paramount in the survival skills of finding food and avoiding becoming food for something else.

Perhaps the most obvious survival skill is the ability to avoid or overcome danger. Our species wouldn't have survived very long if our remote ancestors hadn't been able to get out of the way of, or kill, predators that saw our kind as a tasty link in the food chain. But times have changed. In our society, few of us need be overly concerned about wild animal predators roaming our "urbs" and suburbs. But we still have opportunities to call on our survival instinct to avoid potentially life-threatening modern-day dangers. We can duck, jump, or scramble to get out of harm's way. But if you can't move well, you may not be able to scurry out of the way of a driver who doesn't see you in the crosswalk. Or, you may not be able to duck out of the line of fire of a baseball hurtling toward your head.

WELLNESS PRINCIPLE: You were designed to
survive.

Survival involves more than successfully re-sponding to physical threats from the outside. Your body must survive the things you put into it — tangibles such as food, drink, drugs, and the air you breathe. And, that's not all. Your body must survive your thoughts and attitudes.

The survival concept is very important. When you realize that *every* physiological function of your body is a survival function, you begin to look at health in a different way.

WELLNESS PRINCIPLE: Survival is your body's only
goal.

"If the body is designed to survive," you might be thinking, "why do we have pain, illness, and death?"

That's a good question. It deserves a good answer.

To answer the last part first, we all are going to die sometime. When I say the body is designed to survive, I mean that the purpose of every function of the body is to survive conditions of the present. That concept leads to the pain and illness part of the question.

The body wasn't designed to be healthy. It wasn't designed to be sick.

The body responds instant by instant to the internal conditions it must work with. Inner workings aren't concerned with the long-term consequences of its survival tactics. Internal workings aren't concerned with anything other than survival of conditions of the moment. It's rather like the fellow who jumps into a lake

to escape a swarm of marauding bees. He isn't concerned about
losing his contacts or ruining his new $150 athletic shoes. He
isn't even concerned with the fact that he isn't a good swimmer.
His only concern is survival of the moment.

So it is with internal responses to stimuli from the outside or
inside. Internal responses are automatic and perfect for every
occasion. And you have little control over them.

The inner workings of your body are controlled by your
subconscious. When you sprint for the lake or chop wood, you
don't need to consciously decide that your heart and breathing
will speed up to get more oxygen to your muscles. When you are
frightened, you don't need to consciously put all of your defense
mechanisms on alert. And after you've gorged on Thanksgiving
dinner or nibbled on a snack, you don't need to decide to digest
food. You don't need to instruct your body to repair major or
minor injuries. Everything that goes on inside your body is
automatic and perfect. Every internal response is a subconscious
response to a current condition. And you didn't need to learn
these responses. They were inborn. Or to put it another way, they
were full grown at birth.

WELLNESS PRINCIPLE: Your subconscious never
                      makes a mistake.

All of your internal processes happen without you even
realizing they are going on. Your subconscious communication
systems take care of all of the details. The only purpose of all of
those details is survival of the internal situation of the moment.
Of course, as soon as one detail changes, the situation changes
and different internal conditions must be survived. That's your
body's job. Survive each moment according to the situation or
need.

Survival is the motivation behind any and all physiological
functions. We use the terms "physiological" and "physiology"
frequently in this book. They are short-hand for referring to the

physical, chemical, and electrical activities of living organisms — cells, organs, systems, us. All physiological activity of your body is directed toward surviving internal conditions of the moment. Since those conditions change constantly, your physiology changes constantly. And physiological changes are automatic. You don't control them. You can influence them by the choices you make in the six essentials, but you don't control them.

For example, when you eat or drink *anything*, your physiology changes immediately to handle the threat of new substances in your body. Similarly, when you begin to run, your physiology changes. Cells need more oxygen. Muscles need oxygen to function. The more you use the muscles, the more oxygen they need. Blood carries oxygen. So you breathe faster and harder to take in more oxygen, and your heart pumps faster and harder to deliver the oxygen to cells and tissues.

However, eating and physical effort aren't the only stimuli that affect your physiology. Emotions attached to thoughts affect physiology.

The big difference between eating/exercising and emotions/thoughts is that you eat and exercise only periodically. You think and feel all the time. So thinking is a more constant physiological factor than eating or exercising. Nonetheless, whatever the stimulus and wherever it comes from, your body adapts to survive it and all other stimuli. Anything that requires your body to change what it's doing is a stress.

> WELLNESS PRINCIPLE: Everything you do, feel,
> and think causes stress to
> your body.

CHOICE STRESS

Your body responds to everything that happens to it or is put into it. When you exercise, your body must respond in ways that assure immediate survival of the new activity. Heart rate and blood pressure go up. Digestion decreases. Pupils dilate. Your body is primed to run or fight. That's stress.

We usually think of stress as a negative condition that must be overcome or dealt with. We say we are stressed when bad things happen to us. We become upset, anxious, fearful, angry, or respond with other so-called negative emotions. But as far as your body is concerned, stress is more than emotional upheaval. In body language, *stress is anything that causes a change in the way your body is functioning at the moment.*

Even eating is a stress to your body. You might be enjoying a jolly holiday feast with loved ones and friends and be happy as a mosquito at a nudist camp, but as soon as you put that first bit of food into your mouth, your body is stressed. It must change some of its functions to meet the challenge of new substances in your body. The food must be digested. Your digestive mode gets in gear. That's a physiological change. And physiological change is stress.

However, not to worry. Your body is designed to handle the stress of new food. And it doesn't take any planning or action on your part. You don't have to consciously decide: "Okay, stomach, pump acid. Break down this hamburger I just ate, and don't forget that bit of pickle that came with it." No, your body makes the necessary adjustments without your help. It's all automatic. And, it's all part of the survival game. If your body couldn't switch from not-digesting to digesting, the hamburger — and the pickle — would just sit in your stomach and rot. That's not good.

But what about those things we usually consider stress? Anger, fear, anxiety, and all that?

These emotions also bring about changes in your physiology. Your body prepares itself to defend itself against perceived dangers. I call this "defense physiology," or "survival physiology." Your body gets ready to run or fight. And to do that, it must switch from its ho-hum, everything-is-great mode to danger mode.

WELLNESS PRINCIPLE: Stress is anything that
                                    causes change in the way
                                    your body is functioning.

There's nothing wrong with stress in itself. Stress goes with living. Your health suffers when you inflict inappropriate stress on your body over and over and over. Inappropriate stress, as we shall see, keeps your body in defense even though there is no real and present threat to physical survival. When that happens, your body doesn't have a chance to recoup and repair. Your survival mechanisms are designed to prepare you to get out of short-term life-threatening emergencies — the tiger that's eyeing you as dinner, an out-of-hand fire in the cave, a man coming at you with a gun, or any other threat to life and limb. These are examples of short-term physical threats. They happen, then they're over. It's appropriate for your physiology to be in defense or survival mode.

However, threats such as worry, anxiety, and guilt aren't as clear cut. They may have a clearly defined beginning, but they don't have a neat, well-defined end. Your physiological survival mechanisms never get the all-clear signal, so defense physiology goes on indefinitely. Eventually, overworked organs and systems become exhausted. And exhaustion opens the door to pain and ill-health.

Does that mean that your body is stupid since it can't tell the difference between appropriate and inappropriate threats?

No way.

As far as your body is concerned, a threat is a threat. Any time your emotions signal danger, your subconscious responds with defense. Your subconscious doesn't think, judge, or reason. That's the job of your conscious mind.

WELLNESS PRINCIPLE: Physiological responses to
                                    stress are non-judgmental.

Every response of your body is perfect for the stimulus causing the response. You may not like the response, but it's perfect for your survival whether you like it or not.

THE BODY INTELLIGENT
Our bodies are far more intelligent than we will ever be. They always respond perfectly. Our physiological bodies know exactly how to respond to stimuli, and they don't make mistakes in the response. Oh, that we could say the same for ourselves in our external life.

Sometimes the response is to ignore the stimulus. If you are sitting in a comfortable chair reading at this moment, you are probably not aware of the weight of your body on your buttocks and legs. Now, if you have been sitting on a hard chair for quite a while, you may be extremely aware of the hardness of the chair and your increasingly uncomfortable position.

Yet, even then, you probably aren't aware of the feel on your skin of the clothes you are wearing. At least you weren't until you read this. Many of the stimuli that the body receives are ignored — they are commonly received stimuli and they are not threatening.

More stimuli affect your physiology than those that come from the outside. Internal stimuli keep your nervous systems constantly appraised of conditions inside your body.

Most of us don't think too much about the intricate chemical and electrical processes going on in our inner workings to keep us functioning and reasonably comfortable. Inside your body temperature stays constant, food is processed, nutrients are distributed to cells, messages zip around your nervous systems, organs and systems maintain rhythmic processes, debris is segregated and eliminated, wounds are healed, muscles contract and relax, chemicals are produced — the list goes on. And, for the most part we never give any of it a thought until something gets out of synch. Physiological activity is rather like the electric service to your house: you take it for granted until something calls it to your attention.

WELLNESS PRINCIPLE: Everything your body does
is perfect for survival and
to meet conditions of the
moment.

Your body was designed by an Infinite Intelligence and functions with infinite intelligence. It responds perfectly to every stimulus. Your body is an integrated whole. It "talks" to itself. But your body doesn't think!

This is a difficult concept for many people. How can we say that the body responds perfectly when so many of us are in pain or sick and tired? The general belief is that when things go wrong with health, the body is doing something wrong.

It isn't. Your body never does anything wrong physiologically. You may not like the outcome of its responses, but the internal response is always correct for the stimulus it is responding to. The response is always correct. However, as we said earlier, the stimulus may be inappropriate.

High blood pressure is an example.

Suppose you have just finished a five-mile run. Or, you have spent the afternoon carrying bags of cement. Or, you have just had an animated, high-level disagreement with your boss, spouse, or significant other. If you were to take your blood pressure, it would be higher than "normal" — 160 over 90 instead of a "normal" 120 over 80. You wouldn't find that at all unusual or "wrong." You were exerting yourself, stressed, or up-tight. When the stressful event is over, down goes the blood pressure. No big deal. It went up to help pump more oxygen-containing blood to your muscles, and went down when the muscles no longer required the additional oxygen supply.

Okay. So, we know that your blood pressure can rise and fall depending upon the circumstances.

But suppose you are slouched in front of the TV watching an

uninspiring program. Your mind is in neutral and you are about
as relaxed as you can get.

You take your blood pressure and, again, it's 160 over 90 —
numbers that indicate elevated blood pressure. Now you're
concerned.

Your body isn't doing anything wrong. Elevated blood
pressure is a perfect response. You need for your blood pressure
to be able to go up. However, it doesn't need to be above normal
when you are resting. A stimulus of some sort is signaling the
need for elevated blood pressure. Your body is responding
perfectly to that stimulus even though you're "relaxed." So, the
stimulus is inappropriate, not the blood pressure level.

Your body was designed to do high blood pressure. Your
body can't do anything it wasn't designed to do. It wasn't
designed to fly, so you can't fly. However, everything your body
was designed to do serves a purpose. We may not always
understand the purpose behind every physiological function, but
that doesn't mean there isn't one. Your body doesn't do anything
silly, useless, unnecessary, or just for kicks. Depending on the
stimulus, your body can do a correct function at an inappropriate
time. When your body is performing any physiological function
at an inappropriate time, it's the stimulus that is the problem, not
the physiological function.

WELLNESS PRINCIPLE: Your body never does anything "wrong."

Your body is infinitely intelligent. It is designed to do
everything it needs to do to survive all but the most major
trauma. Does that mean that we are designed to live forever?

Certainly not.

Eventually, cells, organs, and systems "wear out." However,
barring major physical trauma, if we consistently make correct
choices in the six essential areas of life, we have a good shot at
living to a ripe old age and dying peacefully in our sleep rather

than at a young age while running.

Exercise is one the six essentials of life. Exercise is also one of the perks of being alive. It is a vehicle for activity, productivity, fitness, and can be just plain fun. In fact, if exercise doesn't include at least a little pleasure and enjoyment, you're doing the wrong kind and you won't continue it very long.

You can exercise to strengthen muscles, increase endurance, lose weight, and improve your cardiovascular system. But don't expect exercise to make you healthy.

Health, either good or not-so-good, is a whole-body condition. It's more than fitness, strength, stamina, muscles, heart, liver, kidneys, or any one organ or system. Any part of your body affects your whole body. We can treat symptoms that affect particular body parts, but the whole body is affected by both the "problem" and the "treatment." Anyone who has ever taken medicine, had surgery or a stomach ache, been injured, broken a bone, or pulled a muscle (and that includes just about all of us) knows about "side effects." Pain or discomfort may be localized, but its effects radiate throughout the body. Tweak your body in one place, and the whole body responds.

The bottom line is that fitness is fine — if you're healthy. But you don't get healthy by getting fit. You don't get healthy by exercising. Furthermore, if your internal environment isn't reasonably healthy, you shouldn't exercise strenuously.

Health involves more than being fit. It is a by-product of making appropriate choices in the six essential areas of life.

Once you are healthy, exercising toward fitness is fine. But if you aren't into rigorous training, you can still exercise and feel better. We'll go into the most advantageous types of exercise later, but first, we'll take a brief look at the other essentials of life.

CHAPTER 2

THE SIX ESSENTIALS

CHOICE MATTERS
We all eat, drink, breathe, exercise, rest, and think. These are the six essentials of living. And all six are involved in survival.

We must engage in the six essentials just to stay alive. Even exercise is a requirement for survival. Although we generally think of exercise as some sort of physical routine — working out, running, golf, and the like — exercise is movement. Movement is necessary to gather food, find shelter, and take care of yourself. The six essentials are natural functions designed for survival.

The six essentials are different from natural internal functions such as heart beat, insulin production, or peristaltic action of your digestive system. Internal functions are automatic; the six essential areas offer choices. And you make these choices constantly. You choose how, how much, what, where, or when you do them.

We can survive for weeks without eating or exercising. We can manage for several days without drinking or resting. If we put our minds to it, we can go a couple of minutes without breathing. But, like it or not, when we are awake, we think constantly

The six essentials are integral parts of our lives. There's no question whether or not we will eat, drink, think or any of the others. The question is of quality. And quality is a matter of choice. When we consistently make appropriate choices, we give our bodies the opportunity to function smoothly. When we consistently make inappropriate choices, we make our internal functions work harder and adapt to handle stressful situations. Our bodies must adapt and compensate to unnecessary stress. In time, organs and systems become exhausted. Then, the door is open to discomfort, illness, pain, and disease. And, it's all a matter of the choices we have made over long periods of time. If we continue to do what we have always done, we will continue to get the same results.

> WELLNESS PRINCIPLE: Choice is the health factor
> of the six essentials.

Appropriate choices are those that allow your body to function as smoothly as possible for as much of the time as possible. Your body functions smoothly when it handles temporary stress then shifts back into maintenance and repair.

Stress isn't bad. Your body was designed to handle stress. But stress should be a short-term condition. Handle the situation, then back to maintenance and repair. That's the response to appropriate choices — short-term stress responses followed by recovery.

We know that your body has been, is being, and will be stressed. Eating and drinking stress your body. Accidents stress your body. Emotions stress your body. Lack of rest stresses your body. Polluted air stresses your body. Even exercise — movement — stresses your body. But, your body is designed to handle these stresses and other stresses, then get back to business as usual. That's the key to appropriate choices of the six essentials. They are choices that inflict only brief periods of stress on the body from which it can recover quickly.

Inappropriate choices inflict unnecessary or long-term stress on the body. The same inappropriate choices made over and over leave little opportunity for the body to rest, recoup, and recover. Habitual inappropriate choices keep your body responding to the same emergency. It doesn't have time to recover and rest. Organs and/or systems get tired.

The body can handle the stress of the occasional inappropriate choice. Special occasion indiscretions in choices of food, drink, rest, breathing, exercise, and thinking probably won't have a lasting effect on your overall health. However, if the "occasional" becomes "habitual" or constant, the body keeps fighting the same stress battle. And long-term stress leads to exhaustion.

> WELLNESS PRINCIPLE: Inappropriate choices are
>   the biggest contributors to
>   long-term stress.

You have little control over many of the stimuli that bombard your body. External stimuli come from outside your body — sensations from sights, sounds, odors, tastes, and touch. And you have less control over internal stimuli such as electrochemical messages throughout your nervous systems and from muscles and organs. But you can control your "thought" responses to external stimuli and make appropriate choices in the other five essentials to keep your internal environment as stress-free as possible. And since your health is a reflection of the internal environment, your overall health is a reflection of the choices you make in the six essentials.

Everything you do involves at least one of the essentials. When you make appropriate choices in the six essentials most of the time, your body is better able to handle stress with ease. If you consistently make inappropriate choices in any of the six essential areas, your body stays in crisis mode. Eventually organs and systems of your body can become exhausted. And when organs or systems are exhausted, you can't be healthy, no matter how fit or symptom-free you are.

> WELLNESS PRINCIPLE: Health — good or ill — is a
>   whole-body condition.

One of the objectives of this book is to help you understand that proper exercise, rest, and breathing are only part of any health program. You are an integrated being — everything affects everything else. The six essentials are a package deal. This book focuses on the essentials of exercise, rest, and breathing, so we'll take a only brief look at the other three — eating, drinking, and thinking. Since the eating and drinking essentials are hot topics these days, we'll first take a very quick look at those.

THE FOOD ESSENTIAL

The *types* of food you are in the habit of eating are more important to your health than the particular foods you eat. Well, that doesn't hold true for poisonous mushrooms, Salmonella-laced foods, and other life-threatening indelicacies. These are fast-acting toxins. But some more common foods can have a slower toxic effect on the body. The effect is so slow that it's hard to make the connection unless you are aware of the link. That slow-acting, health-inhibiting food is *excess* dietary protein.

If you have been a "lots of muscle-building protein, steak and eggs, and hold the vegetables" sort of person, you are eating *too much* protein. Your body may be working overtime just to survive. If you lean to the vegetarian side as a "pass the pasta, cheese, nuts, and yogurt" sort of person, you still may not be getting the beneficial effects you expect from your diet. Even vegetarians can get too much protein.

"Hold it!" your protein-enculturated thoughts scream. "We need protein. Athletes eat lots of protein to help build muscles. Protein is good!"

And you're right — to a degree.

We do need protein. We don't need *too much* protein in our diets.

Protein is amino acid. We are protein people, and we eat protein. However, we don't need to eat as much protein as most Americans eat. Besides, we get protein from foods other than flesh foods of meat, poultry, and fish. We're talking about more dietary protein than the body needs.

The ideal food choices for your body are those that result in a diet made up of about 70% vegetables and fruits and 30% meats, poultry, fish, grains, and dairy products. The 30% category comes from high-protein food.

> WELLNESS PRINCIPLE: Protein is good; too much
> dietary protein isn't.

You see, it all revolves around the internal environment mentioned earlier. Your internal environment is where your cells live.

When you were born, most of your internal fluids were slightly alkaline. Throughout your life, your intelligent body works to keep them that way. Of course, the fluid in your stomach is highly acid when there's food to be digested. But other than that, the fluids in your body should be just on the alkaline side of neutral. That's the way it's designed to function best.

Before we go into the perils of excess protein, we'll have a short refresher on acid and alkali (or "base" as alkali is sometimes termed). Either strong acid or strong alkali can damage tissue. On the home front, battery acid is strong enough to burn your skin, vinegar is a weaker acid. Oven cleaner is a strong alkali that can burn your skin, ammonia is weaker but still potent, and baking soda is an even weaker alkali. Your body can handle vinegar and baking soda, but battery acid and oven cleaner can cause major damage. Your intelligent body does everything in its power to avoid being damaged by either strong acid or strong alkali. Your body does whatever is necessary to keep acid and alkaline in balance. How does it do that? By neutralizing any strong stuff to make it weaker.

The body keeps its acid/alkaline balance by adding alkaline neutralizers to acid. Add an alkaline substance to acid, and it weakens the acid. You can demonstrate the neutralizing process by a little experiment. Put a teaspoonful of alkaline baking soda in a small glass of acid vinegar and watch the reaction. In the body, the process is equally as effective but much less violent.

Many of the physiological processes in your body are directed toward maintaining a slightly alkaline environment everyplace except in the stomach when there's food to be digested.

Our cells work best in an environment that is slightly alkaline. But many of our choices are acid producers. In addition, acid is produced when cells function, which they do constantly. So your body spends a lot of time and energy keeping itself from getting too acidic. But there's a big difference in the acid that comes from acid-producing foods and the acid your cells generate. Physiological acid from cellular function is eliminated when you breathe. That's the carbon dioxide that you exhale. No big deal.

WELLNESS PRINCIPLE: We are alkaline by design
and acid by function.™

In contrast, dietary acid from acid-producing food is eliminated through the kidneys. You can't just "blow it off." Dietary acid is rather strong. Not super strong like battery acid, but strong for the body. So before it goes through delicate kidney tissue, dietary acid must be neutralized. That's no big deal either, as long as there's not too much. Even though your body is designed to be slightly alkaline, it is also designed to handle moderate amounts of acid on a temporary basis.

Many of the foods we eat leave an acid "after glow." When we talk about dietary acid, generally the first foods that spring to mind are lemons, peaches, grapefruit, oranges, and other fruits. These foods are acid going into your body. Acid from most fruits and vegetables, like the self-produced acid from cellular function, is easily eliminated through the lungs — no undo stress on the body.

When we talk about acid foods, we're talking about high-protein foods that aren't particularly acid when you eat them but, as they are digested, they leave an acid residue.

The acid residue of dietary protein is called ash. Acid ash must be neutralized — weakened; made less acid. When you regularly eat a lot of high-protein foods, a lot of acid is left to be neutralized. That's the job of your alkaline reserve. Your alkaline reserve is part of your body's internal maintenance crew. It's essential for keeping your internal environment within slightly alkaline survival limits. In order for you to survive, your blood must stay within a very narrow range of slight alkalinity. And since your body is designed to survive, it will do anything and everything possible to keep your life-sustaining oxygen-carrying blood within survival range.

Sodium — not salt, which is sodium chloride — is an important mineral of your alkaline reserve. Sodium is instrumental in neutralizing internal acid. But sodium is also involved in other important jobs such as transmitting impulses of nerve and muscle fibers, and secreting different substances of various glands.[2] So if you constantly pour excess protein into your body, a lot of sodium is used to neutralize the acid. Eventually, your readily available supply of neutralizing sodium will run low. Then your body must use other neutralizers, such as calcium, to help neutralize the acid from acid ash-producing foods. And you know where most of your calcium is stored — in bones and teeth. You also know what happens when you lose too much calcium from bones. They become brittle and weak.

Your body will do whatever it takes to keep your blood within the required narrow range of slight alkalinity. Most foods have protein in them. Meats, dairy products, poultry, fish, and grains have a high protein content. If you keep dumping too much acid-producing protein into your body without replenishing needed neutralizing minerals, you'll use up your precious available alkaline reserve. Then your body takes "extraordinary measures" to keep your blood acid level within survival limits. Neutralizing minerals are taken from other jobs in the body to keep your acid level under control. The result is that areas of the body that are less survival-specific suffer. Then we give the resulting symptoms names, such as osteoporosis, arthritis, allergies, or general poor health.

> WELLNESS PRINCIPLE: Brittle bones, achy joints, or runny nose aren't as life-threatening as acid blood.

And there's more. If you knock out its first line of neutralizing defense by continuing to make inappropriate food choices, your body calls on "the home guard" backup system. There's more than one way to neutralize acid.

When available alkaline reserve minerals are in short supply and excess acid-producing protein keeps coming and coming, the body calls on emergency backup systems to neutralize the acid to protect delicate tissues. An indication that emergency neutralizing processes have kicked in is the odor of ammonia in the urine. That's a sure sign of long-term excess dietary protein.

Another indicator is early morning stiffness that diminishes during the day.

Through the night, the body has been cleaning up from the day before. But all of the toxins haven't been eliminated from the body yet. As the day goes on and more toxins are eliminated from the body in urine and feces, we feel better and "limber up."

Many of the discomforts, pains, illnesses, and diseases we suffer can be traced to inappropriate food choices. As a nation, we are heavy into protein. Fortunately, more and more people are beginning to see the benefits of being heavier into vegetables and fruits than they were in the past.

Plant foods contain more of the all-important sodium and other minerals your body needs to function and to neutralize dietary acid. Most fruits and vegetables leave an alkaline ash to offset the acid of acid ash-producing foods and help keep your internal environment slightly alkaline. With a diet of about 70% vegetables and fruits and 30% meat, poultry, fish, dairy products, and grains, you get enough minerals to handle dietary acid plus enough to keep your alkaline reserve well stocked.

WELLNESS PRINCIPLE: Nurture by nature — eat plants.

But a word of caution: If you usually eat a lot of meat, poultry, fish, and grains, don't make a radical shift to an all fruit and vegetable diet. Your body is accustomed to handling your usual diet. A short adjustment period is best to allow your body to adapt to processing large quantities of "good food." It's not that your body can't handle it. It's that you won't like the way you feel during the transition period. The dedicated meat-eater who makes a quick, dramatic change to a more body-friendly vegetable-intense diet has a tendency to experience diarrhea, flatulence, stiff muscles and joints, and a general feeling that ranges from bad to horrible. Initially, he or she definitely doesn't feel better on the new diet. So what happens? After a couple of days of misery, malcontent sets in. They decide that all this "veggies are good for you" is a bunch of health-nut propaganda and they go back to their old way of eating. And of course, the symptoms go away. They may feel better, but they aren't doing their body any long-term favors.

WELLNESS PRINCIPLE: Don't go whole hog on vegetables if you're not used to them.

Improving your diet (and health) by increasing your fruit and vegetable intake works best when you mimic the routine of those who begin eating again after having been without food for long periods. They make the transition slowly. So, let your body ease into a better diet.

Begin by adding one serving of cooked vegetables a day. Cooked vegetables are best if your body isn't accustomed to plant food. After a couple of days, add a second serving of cooked vegetables. Then, in about a week, increase your fruit allotment. When you use the slow and steady method, your body can adjust to the "new foods" without the "dietary distress" that often accompanies an all-out change.

In our society, finding food isn't much of a challenge. We tend to look on eating as recreation and to forget that it is an essential of living and health. The challenge is to make sure that the food you give your body is not only satisfying but supplies the vitamins and minerals your body needs to maintain slight alkalinity. Eating is one of the six essentials. It's the only way we can replenish vital nutrients. Choosing foods that replace the minerals needed to carry out internal functions should be equally as high on your health enhancing priority list as exercise.

WELLNESS PRINCIPLE: Feed your alkaline reserve
as well as your appetite.

DRINKING IS ESSENTIAL

One of the great mysteries of life is why we don't splash and slosh when we move. A 150 lb. man totes around about 42 quarts of water. Water makes up about 57% of our total body weight.[3] For a newborn, water can account for as much as 75% of body weight.[4]

More than half of the fluid in our bodies is inside the cells — intracellular fluid. And we have about 75,000,000,000,000 (that's trillion) cells. The rest of the fluid is outside the cells — extracellular fluid. Extracellular fluid includes interstitial (around cells) fluid, plasma, cerebrospinal fluid, intraocular fluid, fluids of the gastrointestinal tract, and the fluid in spaces where one surface moves against another. These are the fluids we talked about earlier that should be slightly alkaline.

Our supply of fluids isn't constant. We consume them and we lose them. For the most part, we take in fluids through our mouth, although a bit is self-generated. We lose fluids in several ways. The most obvious fluid removal vehicles are urine and the feces. Less obvious, is the moisture that accompanies each breath as we exhale or the diffusion of fluids through the skin, more colorfully described as sweat. In normal temperature conditions, we lose roughly 4.5 pints of fluid a day. More as the temperature outside the body rises or as physical activity increases.

Drinking is essential to replenish the fluids in your body. If you don't replace the fluids your body loses, your body becomes dehydrated. Dehydration reduces extracellular fluid and blood volume. When the fluid and blood volumes go down, less oxygen and fewer nutrients are delivered to cells and tissues.

WELLNESS PRINCIPLE: Replenishing fluids is part
of the survival game.

Ordinarily, we have plenty of opportunities to replenish our fluids. In our commercial society, we have sweet drinks, carbonated drinks, sports drinks, alcoholic drinks, coffee, tea, milk, fruit juice, bottled water, tap water, and more. These are generally pleasant-tasting, meal accompaniments or social drinks. Some of them aren't even thirst-quenchers. In fact, some sweet drinks may offer only temporary relief and leave your thirstier than you were before. The best thirst-quencher is pure water.

Water
"Pure" water is the best between meal drink. But "pure" water is hard to come by these days. We have managed to muddy-up our environment enough so that we don't have "pure" water left. However, along with the technology that has contaminated our water supply, we have technology to clean it up. Most cities and towns have water treatment plants that reduce the pollution of the

water we drink. Unfortunately, the cleaning-up process is done by adding chemicals to the water. Sure enough, chemicals neutralize the health-threatening effects of the microscopic "critters" in the water, but your body really doesn't need those particular chemicals.

The best home-style water purification system uses a reverse osmosis (RO) process. The next best type of water for your body is distilled water with a dash of fresh lemon juice. Distilled water is considered by some to be the most health-enhancing water. Unfortunately, distilling takes all the life out of the water. That's the purpose of the fresh lemon juice — to rejuvenate "dead" water.

Many athletes, and athlete imitators, have turned to sports drinks to replenish the fluids their bodies lose as sweat during strenuous exercise. Sports drinks are designed to replace not only water but also electrolytes. Electrolytes are minerals, such as salts of sodium, potassium, and chlorine, that take on electrical charges and help conduct electric current such as nerve impulses. As Covert Bailey puts it, "They're like little batteries."[5]

However, sports drinks also contain sugar. You can get the same effect of water and electrolyte replacement without the sugar by drinking pure water flavored with fresh, unsweetened fruit juice. Keep in mind that the most ardent advocates of these specialty beverages are the drink manufacturers. If you do high-intensity exercise for long periods, like running or bike riding marathons, you may need to replace electrolytes. Otherwise, water will work. Your body definitely needs water replacement; it *might* need electrolyte replacement.

At meals, the very best "drink" comes in solid form — fruits and vegetables. When your diet is heavy on the fruits and vegetables side, the best kind of water is built into your food. Fruits and vegetables come equipped with fluids that provide both water and nutrients. Most people who make the transition to a vegetable-and-fruit-centered diet find they aren't as thirsty as they were on a meat-centered diet. With vegetable-based meals, you satisfy your thirst as well as your hunger.

When you eat plenty of fruits and vegetables, you don't need to drink as much water as you do when you eat a lot of meat and grains. The traditional eight glasses of water a day is overkill. It probably won't do you any harm, but you don't really need it unless you are thirsty. For most of us, that's the key to knowing how much to drink.

> WELLNESS PRINCIPLE: Your need for fluids
>   depends on your diet.

Milk

We begin our nutritional life with milk. Human mother's milk (of a healthy mother) is the most perfect food for infants. Goat's milk is a poor second, and cow's milk a distant third. Mother's milk contains all of the nutrients a tiny body needs to get going in life. But after a child has teeth and can eat nutritious fruits and vegetables, little (if any) milk is necessary. In fact, great quanti-ties of pasteurized cow's milk can do more harm than good. Pasteurized cow's milk isn't even good for calves. Studies have shown that calves can't survive on pasteurized milk.

> WELLNESS PRINCIPLE: Raw cow's milk is a perfect
>   food — for calves.

Cow's milk has an acidifying effect on the body. Conse-quently, for adults (most of whom already get too much dietary acid), milk can contribute to osteoporosis rather than prevent it. But that's not the sort of thing the dairy industry wants to admit or even hear.

The concept of milk as "nature's nearly perfect food" is so firmly ingrained in our society that parents find it difficult to "deny" their post-toddler children the alleged nutritional value of milk. However, man is the only mammal that continues to drink milk after the weaning age. In addition, many children and adults have adverse reactions to milk. Children and adults who follow a well-balanced diet that includes plenty of vegetables and fruit can get the nutrition they need without the disadvantages of milk.

Fruit and Vegetable Juice

Fruit juice is an excellent fluid replenisher. But like just about everything else in life, when you drink fruit juice, moderation is the key. You don't need too much. Juice is fruit in concentrated form. Drink only as much fruit juice at a time as you would get from eating your fill of the fruit the juice comes from.

Fruit juice gives your body valuable minerals and vitamins. Most commercially prepared fruit juice also gives your body more sugar than you need. When you prepare your own juice from fresh, ripe fruit, you know you aren't getting excess sugar.

With a juicer, you can not only juice fruits, you can juice vegetables for refreshing, nourishing drinks. When juicing vegetables, taste the vegetables before juicing. Use only sweet-tasting vegetables. However, if after juicing, the juice tastes bitter, throw it out in your garden and let nature recycle it.

The underlying principle in making appropriate choices in the drinking essential is to replenish your fluid supply by eating plenty of fruits and vegetables and drinking the purest "live" water you can find.

Eating and drinking are the two most obvious essentials. They have a major impact on your health. We have merely touched on the high spots of how the acid factor affects your internal environment and your health.

Food and drink are very important to your body's survival and smooth functioning. Equally as important are your thoughts, memories, and emotions. Your thinking essential is so important to your health it deserves a chapter of its own.

CHAPTER 3

THOUGHT-FULL PHYSIOLOGY

WHEN IT COMES TO MIND

Thoughts are powerful. Thoughts are behind your major and minor decisions. They guide your life, and they can affect the way your body functions. As a potential health hazard, thought can rank right along with improper diet, lack of exercise, inappropriate drinking, and cigarette smoking.

We give conscious thought to selecting a career or mate. We give at least passing thought to making choices in the six essentials. But, we probably don't give much thought to the effect thinking has on our physiological functions. Thinking about exercising, for example, can increase heart rate and the strength of heart contractions and constrict blood vessels throughout the body. That doesn't mean that thinking about exercising is a substitute for the real thing. It illustrates the power thoughts have over physiology.

The choices you make about how you think and respond to the world and people around you have an equal or greater impact on your long-term health than any or all of the other essentials. But we're not talking about think-lovely-wonderful-thoughts-and-all-will-be-right-with-the-world thinking. We're talking about thoughts, feelings, and attitudes that color your view of yourself, other people, your experiences, and the things that go

on in your life. Your body responds physiologically to feelings
that spring from conscious thoughts.

Depending upon the feelings, internal organs and systems
speed up or slow down. Among the most obvious examples of
this speeding up and slowing down is the connection between
fright and heart rate. Have a good scare, and the physiological
response of your heart can be obvious. However, many other
physiological responses to that scare, or other emotions, are less
apparent. Just because your heart isn't boom-boom-booming
doesn't mean that your physiology is calm and collected.

The following lists describe some common human emotions.
Which of these emotions do you experience frequently?

Do you often feel . . .

Afraid	Apprehensive	Anxious
Angry	Jealous	Resentful
Guilty	Inadequate	Unhappy
Envious	Hopeless	Worthless
Callous	Irritated	Bitter
Hostile	Useless	Ashamed
Isolated	Embarrassed	Worried
Abandoned	Powerless	Victimized
Indecisive	Enraged	Unworthy
Suspicious	Self-contempt	Persecuted
Terror	Depressed	Enraged
Inept	Defeated	Pessimistic

Or, do you more often feel . . .

Creative	Peaceful	Tranquil
Trusting	Confident	Excited
Fulfilled	Self-assured	Hopeful
Cheerful	Stable	Caring
Exuberant	Satisfied	Productive
Energetic	Enthusiastic	Secure
Happy	Friendly	Loved
Loving	Useful	Worthy
Capable	Successful	Optimistic

The types of feelings characterized by the first list we generally call "negative feelings." They stimulate your internal workings so you can run or fight. Stimulating thoughts and feelings hypercharge your internal "engine" and affect either your muscles or digestion.

You need to be "turbo charged" on those occasions when you must defend against threats to your continued existence. Your body goes all out when you perceive a threat to your person. That's good. You need to be able to defend yourself. But, for your health's sake, you don't need to be in defense all the time. That's not only nerve racking, it's exhausting. Besides, the harder your body works, the more acid the cells produce. If your thoughts and feelings keep your body in defense mode constantly, not only do organs and systems work overtime but your internal environment becomes more acid, and your body becomes more toxic. We said earlier that cells produce acid when they function. The harder your body works, the more acid is produced. So, on top of keeping you ready to defend, your body has to work even harder to keep itself slightly alkaline. That's an exhausting combination for any body.

That's what constant negative feelings and thoughts can do to you.

However, pleasant feelings — "positive feelings" as described in the second list — also affect your body. When you are exhilarated and excited, you may feel energetic and ready to jump for joy, but your body isn't geared up to fight. And, as you will see later, the best thing about positive thoughts and feelings is that they don't lock defense-producing emotions into your memory bank.

WELLNESS PRINCIPLE: Thoughts affect your whole
                                              body.

Some thoughts have little impact on your physiology. Your body doesn't get excited when you think something like "Hawaii

became the 50th U.S. state in 1959." Not much of an emotional
wallop there. But you and your body might get quite excited as
you pack to take your first trip to that state. It's the feelings
attached to thoughts that prompt physiological responses. Which
brings us back to survival.

Your body is designed to survive. And how does it do this?
By detecting threatening situations. That's the main purpose of
your five senses — to be aware of threats to your survival. You
see, hear, smell, taste, and feel in order to detect threats that
come at you from the big outside world. Without these senses,
the human race would have died out long before it developed
such technological wonders as cooking fires that doubled as
central heating.

Your five senses are designed to alert you to threats that come
at you from the outside. Your body is designed to make adjustments in the way it is functioning so you can respond to these
threats. As soon as you sense you are threatened, your body shifts
into defense physiology, then you respond to the situation.

WELLNESS PRINCIPLE: Defense physiology
precedes defensive action.

DEFENSE PHYSIOLOGY
Your body is magnificently designed to protect and defend itself.
Yet not all threats come from the outside. Your body is a fortress
that adjusts internal functions to maintain slight alkalinity and a
consistent temperature, ward off or kill microscopic invaders,
repair damage, and take care of round-the-clock maintenance of
normal wear and tear.

Even at your most relaxed, your body defends against threats
to its survival. Your skin, mucous, and tiny hair-like structures
protect you from harmful microscopic invaders. Strong acid in
your stomach helps to kill harmful bacteria that may have slipped
into your body along with the food. White cells in your blood
gobble up unwanted or harmful microorganisms, and your

elimination system sends waste products out of your body. Everything your body does has a purpose.

Your body comes equipped with a vast array of defense mechanisms. The "mechanical" systems of skin, white cells, and stomach acid are just a small part of the tip of the defense system iceberg. Less obvious defense systems are the electrochemical responses to internal signals, such as rising acid levels, and external stimuli, such as the screech of a smoke alarm. Your defense systems are ready to react in an instant, and you rarely (if ever) give the process a first or second thought. For one thing, you're completely unaware of your body's strategies and tactics in lowering your internal acid level. And, for another, we take for granted the noticeable physical responses to potential danger. For example . . .

Suppose you are dozing in your favorite chair when your smoke alarm begins to blare. One instant you are in a blob-like state: mind in neutral, eyes closed, heart puttsing along at a resting rate, blood pressure about as low as it goes; digestive tract processing remnants of a pre-snooze snack; organs and systems leisurely functioning; muscles just hanging around. Then, ALARM! In the next instant all changes. Your defense mechanisms jump into high gear. Eyes open, pupils dilate. Heart rate and blood pressure shoots up. Digestion comes to a halt. Muscles tense. Organs and systems adjust for battle. You're primed. You may be momentarily confused, but you are ready to fight or run — whatever it takes. That's defense physiology. And you didn't give any of the physiological changes a moment's thought. They all happened instantaneously and automatically, compliments of your subconscious mind.

> WELLNESS PRINCIPLE: Defense physiology is an
> immediate response of your
> subconscious mind.

Your subconscious is in full control of the hundreds of

internal functions that keep you alive and on an even keel. Confusion and indecision may reign consciously during the first moments of an emergency, but your subconscious is never confused. Your subconscious knows innately exactly how to adjust your physiology for every crisis. When a threat is recognized, your subconscious marshals all of its defense forces for quick decisive action, rapid oxygen refueling for stronger muscles, and heightened perceptions. Organs that aren't needed for defense are throttled down to allow energy to be focused where it will do the most good. In general, the processes of all of your organs or systems either speed up or slow down when your body confronts a crisis. That's defense physiology.

> WELLNESS PRINCIPLE: Defense physiology is great for survival — it's not necessary when you are out of harm's way.

SUBCONSCIOUS RESPONSE
We like to think we are in control. And, much of the time, we are. We can control our responses to the world around us and the choices we make in the six essentials. But we can't directly control internal physiological responses. Areas of your brain that operate below consciousness — your subconscious — take care of those.

Many of your body's physiological responses, including defense physiology, are controlled by a small portion of your brain known as the hypothalamus. When you are frightened, angry, or otherwise emotionally upset, your hypothalamus is one of the first to know. As soon as it is alerted, it sets off a series of internal events designed for protection. The hypothalamus might be termed the seat of emotions.

Emotions follow perceptions and thoughts. Different thoughts and emotions have different effects on your body. For example, the face pales in intense fear and flushes in anger. However, most

of the effects of emotions can't be seen. They involve internal
organs.

WELLNESS PRINCIPLE: Emotions and thoughts
spark physiological
changes.

Autonomic Nervous System

Organs either intensify or subdue their functions according to the
emotion involved. These changes in intensity are controlled by
the hypothalamus through the autonomic nervous system (ANS)
— one of your several nervous systems.

You have no direct control over your autonomic nervous
system. That's what autonomic means: self-controlling; functioning independently. You should be grateful you don't need to
worry about dilating or constricting your pupils, increasing or
decreasing your heart rate or blood pressure, producing more or
less insulin, increasing or decreasing gastrointestinal activity. If
you had to think about all of those things, you'd never get the
combination right to handle an emergency. Or, on the less
dramatic side, just imagine how your golf game would suffer. If
you had to coordinate all of your internal processes, you
wouldn't have time to think about keeping your head level, your
backswing smooth, and your follow-through complete.

WELLNESS PRINCIPLE: Your ANS is an automatic
labor-saving device.

Like all well-organized entities, your ANS assigns responsibility for carrying out operational details to "middle management" divisions. Two of the most important divisions are the
sympathetic system and parasympathetic system. These terms
may sound intimidating, so a little clarification is in order.
However, since this isn't a physiology text, we'll oversimplify
their missions.

In general, the sympathetic system speeds up organ functions, and the parasympathetic system slows them down. Now please note that I said *in general*. There are exceptions to this rule. However, for our purposes we'll say that sympathetic speeds up and parasympathetic slows down.

This speeding up and slowing down is important for balance. Your body works toward maintaining balance — homeostasis; dynamic equilibrium; respond and return to normal. Speeding up and slowing down are both necessary to handle the various stimuli that bombard your body. But unremitting speeding up or slowing down can affect your health in ways you probably won't like.

WELLNESS PRINCIPLE: Sympathetic speeds; parasympathetic slows.

Sympathetic Responses
The sympathetic system handles jobs such as increasing sweat production, muscle strength, heart rate and contraction strength, blood coagulation, adrenaline secretion, pupil size, and mental activity. At the same time, the sympathetic system inhibits gastric secretions, decreases kidney output, bowel activity, and blood flow to the skin. Sympathetic responses aren't universally "speeded up" responses. Your body doesn't need to be concerned with digesting food or eliminating waste while a hungry tiger is nipping at your heels. The sympathetic system gets you ready for the fast action needed to handle physical danger.

Parasympathetic Responses
But your body doesn't need to run in action mode all the time. So, the parasympathetic system inhibits action mode functions and controls the internal involuntary activities necessary for non-threatening living. The parasympathetic system slows heart rate and decreases the force of cardiac contractions. It also constricts pupil size, allows food to be digested, processed, and eliminated,

and controls body temperature and the secretion of some hormones.

We need to be able to adjust to every condition of every moment. However, we don't need to have either our sympathetic or parasympathetic systems dominate our physiology all the time. Both of them respond to emotions or feeling. And either sympathetic or parasympathetic can dominate if we constantly choose inappropriate thought patterns.

Your sensory perceptions, conscious mind, and subconscious mind work together as a team to handle information about the outside world. You need to be able to identify threats when they come along. And you need to be able to combat them, then return to relative peace and quiet. You don't need to respond constantly to threats that aren't actual threats to your physical safety.

How does your conscious mind identify threats?

Through your five senses.

MAKING SENSE
We perceive the world around us through our five senses.

Our five senses allow us to enjoy the finer things in life — the visual beauty of nature, sounds of stirring music, pleasing tastes of foods, the feel of a soft caress, exciting aromas. Our senses add breadth and depth to living. But that's not their primary purpose. The number one job of our five senses is to detect immediate threats to our physical survival. Everything else they do is icing on the cake.

Our five senses — sight, hearing, taste, touch, and smell — are vital parts of our survival system. They act as early warning systems as they pick up clues to danger — our physiological equivalent of radar. Our senses scan our surroundings and send signals of outside conditions to the conscious mind.

> WELLNESS PRINCIPLE: Our five senses are for sur-
> vival first; enjoyment is a
> perk.

Like radar, a variety of "interference blips" show up on your sensory receiving screen, better known as your conscious mind. But your conscious mind does more than receive; it interprets. It's up to your conscious mind to analyze and make sense of the radar "blips" it receives. Does that visual "blip" indicate a threat? Is that long, mottled brown, crooked, rod-like thing you nearly stepped on a stick or a snake?

If your conscious mind immediately interprets the signal as a snake, your subconscious automatic defense response clicks in so fast that you jump or freeze first and analyze later. Similarly, you respond immediately to a sudden loud noise or an unexpected flash of bright light. Your subconscious defense mechanisms prepare your whole body to fight or run before your conscious mind has a chance to sort out the details. Until your conscious mind determines that a stimuli is harmless, defense physiology kicks in for the fleeting instant tenseness that accompanies a startling sound, sight, aroma, or feeling.

Your subconscious adjusts appropriate internal processes to allow you to address the situation. In the stick-snake example, only a fraction of a second is needed for your subconscious to respond with the fear response to your conscious perception of a "snake." But your conscious mind is still analyzing. If the conscious reinterprets the "snake" as a snake, threat signals continue. If reinterpretation decides it's a stick, the subconscious sounds the "all clear" and calls off the threat response. That's part of the survival package — assume a threat until your conscious mind determines otherwise. The sensory-conscious-subconscious sequence reverberates throughout your waking life. The pattern is so natural it doesn't get a moment's thought.

WELLNESS PRINCIPLE: A crisis is a crisis until
                      proved otherwise.

THE REAL THING
As far as your subconscious is concerned, there is no difference

between a "real" crisis and an "imagined" crisis. A "real" crisis is detected through one or more of your five senses. The screech of the smoke alarm is a "real" crisis. "Imagined" crises originate in conscious thoughts and interpretations. An "imagined" crisis may be extremely upsetting, but it doesn't present a threat to your physical safety. Business problems and family turmoil may be disturbing, but they usually aren't life-threatening.

> WELLNESS PRINCIPLE: We can concoct or sustain
> threats of "imagined" crises.

"Imagined" crises bring on physiological changes similar to those caused by real, life-threatening crises, but, often, not as intense. "Imagined" crises can be sustained by internal feelings, emotions, and memories that "lurk in the shadows of your mind." Typical "imagined" crises that your body responds to are guilt, remorse, shame, and their compatriots. These "crises" may be brought about by memories of bleak happenings in the past. Or, the "imagined" crisis may be worry, fear, anxiety, and the like brought about by thoughts of some catastrophe that might happen in the future.

The problem with imagined crises is that they last a long time. They have no clearly defined end. Your body is designed to handle the "quick and dirty" physical threat of a real crisis. Your physiology rises to the occasion, then returns to normal. With imagined crises, your body rises to the occasion and stays up and ready for a fight indefinitely. That's exhausting.

You were designed to handle short-term threats to your physical survival. But non-stop defense physiology that comes from imagined threats wears down both you and your body.

> WELLNESS PRINCIPLE: A real crisis is a threat to
> survival; an imagined crisis
> is a threat to your health.

Short-Term Threats

Physical threats are short-term stress. An up-close and personal encounter with a hungry tiger doesn't last long. There are only three possible outcomes: you escape; you kill the tiger; or the tiger kills you. No matter which, the incident is over in a matter of minutes. And, if you're still alive, once the threat has passed, your body shifts from emergency-survival mode to maintain-repair mode.

Hungry tigers may not roam our supermarket hunting grounds, but physical-threat emergencies still crop up.

Back to the smoke alarm for a moment. When it goes off, your sense of hearing transmits signals you interpret as danger. Your body responds immediately. It gets ready to fight or run. If you smell or see smoke, two or three senses are picking up threat signals. Survival is threatened. Defend. Your heart pumps blood faster. Your breathing is faster and deeper. Your nervous system is alert.

You don't need to think about increasing your heart rate or any of the other physiological preparations to take action. Your body is primed automatically. After the initial alarm, it's your job to decide consciously whether the threat is real or not — is there a fire, or is the smoke alarm just sounding off?

If the threat is real, you and your body stay in survival defense mode and do what needs to be done. If it's a false alarm, or when the danger is over, your physiology soon returns to its pre-threat condition. That's how physical threats from outside your body are handled. You detect the threat. You and your body respond. When it's over, you and your body relax. There's a beginning, middle, and end. Short-term.

> WELLNESS PRINCIPLE: Your body is designed to handle short-term threats detected through your five senses.

Short-term physical threats may be temporarily tiring, but your body recovers quickly. Long-term threats from inappropriate stress we talked about earlier exhaust both you and your body. So, where do long-term threats of inappropriate stress come from?

Thoughts and memories.

Long-Term Threats

Long-term threats keep internal alarm bells clanging. In some areas of our country and the world, people live with constant threats of physical danger. Violence-prone gangs. Random drive-by shootings. Terroristic bombings. Civil upheavals. Family violence. However, for most of us in this country, threats to life and limb are not the primary health inhibitor. Thought-threats are a more insidious danger to our health. Worry, anxiety, fear, guilt, hate, depression, or the other types of emotions shown in the first list at the beginning of this chapter are the most prevalent thought-threats. For most of us, internal alarms are set off by our own "stinkin' thinkin'" rather than by external threats of physical danger. And our thoughts are always with us.

> WELLNESS PRINCIPLE: Thoughts and memories
> can be rampaging tigers
> that never quit.

We said earlier that physiology can change just by thinking about exercising. Thoughts about exercise are essentially emotionally-neutral. If thinking about exercising can change physiology, just imagine how it is affected by negative thoughts which pack an emotional wallop. Most of us don't dwell on exercise thoughts. But worry, anxiety, hate, rage, and all of those other negative emotions are another matter. When we are upset, negative emotions tend to be full-time companions. They are constant. They keep your body geared for defense. But there's no tiger coming at you. Nothing that you can run from or kill.

Thoughts and memories that act as threat signals have a beginning and a middle, but no end. So your body stays in physiological defense for days, weeks, or years. That's exhausting.

Organs and systems need rest. When they are in crisis mode constantly, eventually they become exhausted and they can't do their best work. And since the body is an integrated whole, when one part is "sick and tired," the whole body is affected. That's why thoughts, memories, and attitudes can affect health. They can keep the body in non-stop defense physiology — and it's all automatic.

> WELLNESS PRINCIPLE: Internal exhaustion is the fast-track to pain and ill-health.

YOUR SIXTH SENSE

Every second, your brain receives thousands of bits of information from the outside world through your five senses. Most of these signals are ignored most of the time. Although your brain receives sensory information about the feel of clothing on your skin, unless something is amiss, your brain doesn't pay any attention to it. It also receives and ignores sensory signals such as the hum of machinery and appliances, the feel of your own weight on the soles of your feet, extraneous conversations of office mates, leaves rustling in the breeze, views of familiar furniture in familiar surroundings. The brain filters out stimuli that are routine, non-threatening, or of little interest.

As the conscious mind receives and filters signals of external happenings, the subconscious receives and responds to signals of internal happenings. Internal messages flit around your body to keep physiological functions under control.

And as if that weren't enough, other signals and communications bounce around the brain. Memories. Memories are self-generated stimuli to which the subconscious responds.

Memories can spark subconscious physiological responses in

the same way as signals from the five senses. And the brain is constantly stimulated by memories. So much so that we can call memories our "sixth sense."

Records of past experiences are stored as electrical patterns in the maze of nerve fibers of the brain. Every current perception is compared with electrochemical records of similar past perceptions and evaluated accordingly. That's why the conscious mind doesn't get excited about the hum of the refrigerator or placement of the furniture. However, if new incoming signals don't fit the memory record of the hum or furniture placement, the conscious mind notices that something is not quite right.

Memory records allow you to read these words. As you read, your conscious mind searches through memory records that can decipher and make sense of these little black squiggles that we call letters and words. The patterns of Chinese writing don't mean a thing to you unless you have established appropriate memory patterns that can be retrieved and used to decode the characters.

WELLNESS PRINCIPLE: Knowledge is retrievable
electrochemical connec-
tions.

Strong emotions are a glue that "sticks" experiences in memory. Emotion attached to an experience helps to glue the *interpretation* of that experience into memory. And we have said that physiology responds to emotions. So when "the facts" of an event are stored in memory, the pattern for the physiological response prompted by the event is also stored. Do you get a headache or backache when you're stressed? Or nauseous before you make a presentation or speak to a group? If these are consistent symptoms for similar occasions, you can pretty well bet that they are patterns for physiological responses stored in memory. Whether or not you consciously recall a previous similar occasion, your subconscious does. It recalls the event, the emotions, and the physiology.

WELLNESS PRINCIPLE: Emotions are the "super
                     glue" that hold memories
                     of events and physiology
                     together.

When the memory pattern of an experience is stimulated, the
attached memory pattern for the physiological response is also
stimulated. And the interesting thing is that you don't even need
to consciously recall the original experience. All that's needed to
reactivate a memory pattern is to stir about in the brain area
where the experience and response patterns are stored.

We all experience taking a spontaneous trip through related
memories to come up with an off-the-wall connection. Your
mind's eye clicks through a sequence of loosely connected
thoughts. You may hear a song that reminds you of high school
graduation. That leads you to think of your best buddy who went
into the army. Army brings to mind Uncle George, the drill
sergeant. Uncle George taps into the ridicule he called "kidding"
that he heaped on you when you were young. You were embar-
rassed and hurt by his "kidding." Now, every time "Uncle
George" pops into your mind, the feelings of embarrassment and
humiliation are retrieved and your physiology responds. Your
physiology clicks into "hurt and humiliation response," and it
happens just by hearing a familiar song of the past.

WELLNESS PRINCIPLE: Strong feelings from way
                     back can affect physiology
                     now.

What do memories have to do with health, exercise, and the
six essentials?

If memories keep your body primed for defense, how is your
body going to relax enough to rest and recuperate properly?

If your physiology is stuck in the "fright" response, forcing muscles to exercise will be counterproductive.

If you are stuck in the "flight" response, how can your food be digested properly?

Everything affects everything else.

Memories signal your subconscious to respond to conditions that no longer exist. Memory is ever active. Your body doesn't care where stimulating signals come from. It doesn't care if the signals are appropriate or not. Your body doesn't think; it responds for survival to the stimuli it receives. If memory stimuli require a defensive response, you get defensive.

WELLNESS PRINCIPLE: The body doesn't do reality
                                         checks on stimuli.

Memories can have a major impact on health. If memories keep your body in defense when defense isn't necessary, some organ or system is going to get very tired. And when an organ or system gets tired enough, symptoms appear. Then you can put a scientific name on it and try to treat it. But you don't need to wait until your health begins to suffer to relieve your body of the need to respond constantly to thought-threats stored in memory.

"Sure," you say. "What do you want me to do? Erase all of my unpleasant memories?"

Not at all.

You can't erase memories without physical damage to your brain. But you can *neutralize* the effects of past unpleasant events that may be undermining your health and energy. You do that by a conscious thought exercise. This is one of the most important exercises for health you can do. Sometimes it's more strenuous than physical exercise. It's called Find-the-Good Exercise. Every experience you have is an opportunity for you to learn a lesson. The lesson may be a very practical how-to lesson: how to build a better birdhouse, or how to get from Albuquerque to Zanzibar. Or, the lesson may be a concept, an idea, or a rule to live by. It might be to learn not to make the same mistakes over and over. Or, that you can't control everything that happens to you, but that you can control how you respond.

> WELLNESS PRINCIPLE: Life's lessons happen *for* you, not *to* you.

Adopting the lesson format for living helps you to salvage enough positive from every experience to neutralize the defense physiology response attached to your memories of those experiences. As a result, your internal systems have opportunities for well-deserved rest, internal toxicity is reduced, and your internal environment improves.

You can't alter your past. But you can control your current thoughts about past trauma and bitter experiences. When you take control of your thoughts, you go a long way toward taking control of your health.

Physical exercise is one aspect of health control. We need to exercise our physical parts to maintain overall health. You consciously control the quantity and quality of your exercise. You can also control your thoughts. You can decide to maintain a death grip on a grudge against anyone who has wronged you. You can decide to take offense at every opportunity. Or, you can decide to find something good in every situation. The objective is to choose thoughts that allow your body to function as easily and as smoothly as possible so that exercise will be beneficial rather than lethal.

We all have ups and downs in our lives. That's part of living. Your thought patterns don't assure a trauma-free life or that you'll never again become angry, frustrated, or emotionally bruised. But your thought patterns do determine *how long* negative experiences affect your physiology. Your thoughts and emotions help you to survive. And your thoughts and emotions can be hazardous to your health.

CHAPTER 4

MORE THAN A MEMORY

INTRODUCING NON-CONSCIOUS

Science has named the physical structures of the brain. The cerebrum, with its cortex that receives sensory information, is the higher level, rational, "seat of learning," thinking part of the brain. This is the area that dominates in the process of conscious thought.

Physically beneath the large hemispheres of the thinking cerebrum are the structures that handle physiology, homeostasis, and the internal management of the body. The thalamus, hypothalamus, cerebellum, and other structures function subconsciously.

The spinal cord, the most primitive level of the CNS, is located even lower physically. The spinal cord also functions below consciousness and can be described as the principle information highway between brain and body. The integrated function of these three levels of the central nervous system make life and movement possible.

The human brain and central nervous system are so complex that even the experts may never fully understand exactly how they work. However, we have ample evidence of the products of their labors. One product of the brain is the ability to learn. We learn from experiences which store specific response patterns in memory. When stimulated, these memory response patterns can excite conscious thoughts, physiological emotions, and physical actions. For example, a pattern of signals tells the subconscious it's time for skeletal muscles to relax or contract to accomplish a specific purpose. The intent to move comes from conscious thought. The stimuli to move muscles come from the subconscious. However, directions for the pattern the muscles follow come from another source. I call this source the non-conscious.

Conscious movement is possible through cooperation of conscious, subconscious, and non-conscious. The subconscious responds to the intent of the conscious and non-conscious.

When we are extremely frightened, physical and physiological responses are survival oriented. Survival is under the direction of the subconscious. When we intend to write a letter or swing a baseball bat, the activity is initiated by the conscious. However, the learned pattern for carrying out the physical movement is provided by the non-conscious.

> WELLNESS PRINCIPLE: The subconscious responses
> are inborn; conscious and
> non-conscious responses are
> learned.

Non-conscious response patterns are developed. They are learned by doing and stored in memories. Memories of learned muscle movement aren't acquired the same way as memories of facts such as your address or phone number. Memories for patterns of learned muscle movement are stored either by repetition or by being "glued" with strong emotions.

Muscles can move without intent. Muscles of a newborn move — arms and legs flail, torso bends and stretches. But flailing-arm muscle movements aren't intellectually inspired, intentional, or productive. Intentional, purposeful movement, such as crawling, walking, and drinking from a glass must be learned by repetition. With repetition, the patterns of nerve impulses that direct particular muscle responses are stored as a non-conscious memory.

To illustrate the principle of non-conscious development, think about a child learning to walk. It's a trial-and-error process. First comes balance. Then comes purposeful, but shaky, forward propulsion. It's an exciting time for parents and child alike. And what is the child doing? Repeating the same movements again and again. (For simplicity, we'll designate the child a she.) When she is about a year old, she has gained some control of her body. She isn't controlling her muscles — that's not a conscious activity. She learns by consciously trying to copy what she has seen others do. Her first steps are tentative. No confident stride with arms swinging. Arms must be used for balance. Uneven surfaces bring falls. But each attempt is more sure than the previous. Her nervous system and musculoskeletal system are becoming better coordinated. She keeps practicing and practicing. As she becomes more skilled, she can run, jump, and turn cartwheels. The wonderful thing is that once learned, the movements are automatic. No more concentrating step by step. And, barring severe trauma, once mastered, the process doesn't need to be relearned. It's all stored in non-conscious memory. The intention to walk is a conscious activity. The subconscious directs muscle activity. The precise pattern for the muscles to follow is stored in non-conscious.

WELLNESS PRINCIPLE:　　Patterns to carry out
learned muscle movements
are stored in non-conscious
memory.

The ability to move intentionally doesn't come fully-developed with the basic subconscious survival package. It's learned through repetition. Nevertheless, once learned, intentional movement, such as walking and talking, isn't something you have to think about consciously. When you decide to thread a needle or scratch your head, the decision is a conscious act, but the pattern of muscle movements needed to carry out the motion comes from non-conscious memory that fulfills your intention. You have learned to coordinate particular muscle movements "without thinking."

Physiological changes necessary to carry out the movements — how fast and how far muscles contract and relax — are directed by the subconscious. Subconscious responses are inborn and perfect. Non-conscious movements are learned, intended responses activated by conscious thought.

> WELLNESS PRINCIPLE: The conscious mind learns;
> non-conscious records; sub-
> conscious executes.

You can see that much of your daily activity is directed by your non-conscious. And you can also see that non-conscious memory plays a major role in many exercise programs. Aerobic exercises, for instance.

Off you go to your first aerobics class and the instructor demonstrates a vigorous dance step set to music. Your job is to imitate that dance step. While you are learning (storing the movements in your non-conscious memory), you must think about what your arms, legs, and torso are supposed to be doing at a particular time. After you have practiced a few times, you don't need to concentrate as hard on the process and you can add speed and vigor to the steps. You have stored the patterns for muscle movement in your non-conscious.

Where is this non-conscious area of the brain located? You won't find it labeled in an anatomy book illustration of the brain. Structures of the brain can be shown as separate components. Your non-conscious isn't a structure. It's a function. It is a coordination of the many elements of the brain we generally think of as being conscious and subconscious.

WELLNESS PRINCIPLE: Non-conscious is function,
not a structure.

RED, GREEN, AND YELLOW

The non-conscious isn't a structure of the brain like the cerebral cortex or cerebellum. To illustrate this elusive but powerful non-conscious, I use the familiar diagram of the structure of the brain with its ridges and furrows to represent the conscious, subconscious, and non-conscious connection. The illustration of the brain on the cover of this book has been colored to show areas that *represent* conscious, subconscious, and non-conscious. Keep in mind that this illustration is not a precise representation of the physical structure of the brain. It is intended to help clarify the concept of conscious, subconscious, and non-conscious as used in this book.

In the illustration, the thin outer covering of the cerebrum — the cerebral cortex — is colored red and represents the "conscious" functions of the brain. That's where most interpretations of sensory signals, analytical and rational (or not so rational) thought originates. I call this area the "Red." Everything in the Red is learned. We use Red information to respond to every situation and to run our lives. That's good. The problem with the Red is that everything we learn isn't always correct. The Red is very powerful, but it can function with faulty information and can make mistakes.

WELLNESS PRINCIPLE: Your Red runs — or ruins
— your life.

The subconscious, particularly the hypothalamus, is represented as a small green area at the lower part of the brain. I call the subconscious the "Green." You have no direct control over your Green. It came fully-equipped and perfect at birth. Every response of the Green is perfect. The Green never makes a mistake. Your personal Green is your direct connection to all of the perfection of Universal Energy. No matter how hard you try, you can't improve it. As long as you live, Green responses are perfect.

WELLNESS PRINCIPLE: Your Green runs your body
perfectly.

The non-conscious that includes your many memories of events and movements is shown in yellow as the largest area. You guessed it; I call that the "Yellow." And the reason it is shown as the largest is that the Yellow non-conscious is a major factor in health and success. That's what this book is all about — health and success and the role of exercise in both.

Your Yellow is responsible for your ability to move purposefully. And, more important, your Yellow may be the original source of chronic or occasional, non-traumatic aches and pains.

WELLNESS PRINCIPLE: Yellow is the memory of
Red learned behavior
coupled with perfect Green
responses.

The red-green-yellow color scheme used to represent conscious, subconscious, and non-conscious was quite accidental. Those were the colors of the markers near at hand when I originally colored a sketch of the brain. However, many of my patients have found that the color representations are more helpful than conventional scientific terms in understanding how the body works and how they can improve their choices in the six essentials. They quickly learn that becoming angry, or harboring guilt are Red-based choices. They also come to understand that chronic indigestion or back pain can be legitimate physiological responses to long-standing Yellow-based memory. And they become more tolerant of pain or distress when they realize that Green responses to both Red and Yellow are always perfect.

For much of this book, we focus on conscious and subconscious activity. However, your Yellow is a major influence on your life and health. Everything in your Yellow is a learned response. These aren't just how-to-ride-a-bike responses. They are also emotional responses. We learn how to respond to different situations. We may learn by watching other people's responses. Or we may learn by trying different responses and settling on the one that gives us the greatest pleasure or payback. Once learned, non-conscious Yellow responses are very powerful. They can override conscious responses and create inappropriate conditions the body must survive. I call this Yellow override.

WELLNESS PRINCIPLE: Learned responses can override survival responses.

YELLOW OVERRIDE
A few of years ago on one of my trips to Europe, I met a patient whose symptoms were a perfect example of Yellow override. A "middle aged," successful businessman who had been very athletic and an avid tennis player could now walk only with the support of crutches. When he stood, his leg muscles were very relaxed. The muscles were rather strong, but so relaxed that he was very unsteady on his feet. When he was lying down, his leg muscles were flabby to the touch. However, when I pressed down on a muscle as little as a quarter of an inch, I found it to be very tense. So here he was, muscles relaxed when they should have been contracted, and contracted when they should have been relaxed. Both walking and sleeping were difficult. He was tired. And he hurt.

I had learned a little about this patient before I met him. For one thing, he had had a very favorable response to radiation therapy for cancer. Since then he had resumed his active, athletic lifestyle. According to his medical doctors, he had no signs of recurring cancer. The leg weakness had come on two or three years after his cancer treatment. He needed crutches to walk and ankle supports to keep his feet from flopping down and tripping him when he took a step. He had seen several prominent medical doctors in Canada and Europe about his leg problems. They couldn't find a medical reason for the weakness or pain and told him to exercise to keep the limited mobility he had.

I examined him as he lay on his back on the examining table. I found that his muscles were so tense that I couldn't easily move his feet more than a few inches apart. I put my hands under his heels and lifted his legs expecting him to bend at the hips. But not this patient. Not only did his legs come up from the table, but his whole torso followed. From his neck down, his muscles were so tight that his body was rigid. That didn't make sense. When he was lying down his muscles were so tense his body was rigid, but when he was standing, his muscles were so relaxed he had to support himself to keep from falling.

How could this be? Since every response of the body is perfectly correct, why were this fellow's muscles contracted when they should have been relaxed, and relaxed when they should have been contracted? As he rested on the examining table, he thought he was relaxed. He said he "felt" relaxed. But he wasn't.

"Something" was giving his Green subconscious information and the Green was responding perfectly. There was nothing wrong with the response; the Green was getting a proper stimulus at an inappropriate time.

As we shall see, he didn't have a "muscle problem." His muscles weren't doing anything wrong. All muscles can do is contract or relax on cue. He had a timing problem. His muscles were responding correctly, but the condition in his life that had initiated the stimuli no longer existed. The stimuli were occurring at an inappropriate time. His perfect Green was getting outdated signals from his Yellow.

WELLNESS PRINCIPLE: In health, as in exercise,
                                            timing is everything.

This patient's symptoms were a classic example of Yellow override. The "something" behind his physical problems was stimuli from his non-conscious. The stimuli were from memories of a particularly upsetting situation he believed in his conscious mind he had "dealt with" long ago. He told me that he believed the incident no longer bothered him. He said he thought about it occasionally, but he no longer dwelled on it. His initial anger and frustration had all but disappeared. However, the memories of the event, the emotions, and the physiological responses were firmly fixed in his Yellow. Non-conscious memories stored by strong emotions were dominating his physiology. His example demonstrates how Yellow override can affect health. His health was in such a state that it was affecting his whole life. He didn't just hurt. He was virtually incapacitated. No longer could he do the things he was accustomed to doing or that he enjoyed doing.

WELLNESS PRINCIPLE: Yellow override can affect
                      your life and your health.

Before I go on with the story of this patient, I must emphasize an important point.

This patient's pain and suffering were not "all in his head." He was in acute physical pain. It was very real. He had followed the proper course of health care in investigating his problem. He had been examined and treated by reputable, capable medical doctors who had found no medical reason for his problems. That doesn't mean that he was "crazy" or "brought it on himself." His pain was real and muscles and tendons were involved.

So, what happened?

I told the patient to answer "yes" or "no" to a question without telling me any of the particulars. The question was: "Did anything particularly upsetting happen in your life about six months before your symptoms began?" His answer was an immediate "yes." I instructed him to think about the situation. His muscle tone changed immediately. The change in muscle tone confirmed that the "cause" of his physical problems was Yellow override.

When he saw that his thoughts brought about a physical response, he insisted on telling me what he had been thinking about. It was a failed business partnership in which he felt he had been betrayed and compromised by his former partner. He had been extremely angry at the time. Now, although he had "handled" the situation in his Red, his Yellow still harbored the information that caused his body to respond with "pre-handled" physiology.

Once the cause of his problem was determined, I helped him update the inappropriate internal signals that had kept his body ready to fight.

But how could his body be ready to fight when the muscles were weak?

That's exactly the point. Internal "threat" messages were constantly "telling" his muscles to be prepared to run or fight. These messages had been non-stop since the upsetting incident. His muscles had been responding to the "threat" messages day-in and day-out, night-in and night-out for years. When he slept, these messages kept his muscles ready to do battle. But time had taken its toll. His muscles were weak because they were tired. Worn out. Exhausted. They were trying their best to follow instructions, but they just couldn't maintain the required fight-or-flight tone any longer.

His muscles that were tense were still responding. They just hadn't reached the complete exhaustion stage — yet. If he had gone on much longer, those muscles would also become flabby. His skeletal muscles would have been virtually useless. He would have continued to "waste away." All of his energies would have been devoted to keeping his internal organs going. You see, his heart and lungs were strong. His internal organs weren't having as severe a problem. They were still strong. Survival depends more on internal organs than on skeletal muscles. And the whole purpose of physiology is survival.

WELLNESS PRINCIPLE: The body's motto: Survival
                                  at any cost.

After several treatment sessions, the patient was greatly
improved. Although he still needed crutches to walk, he could
stand without them. He could go up and down stairs more easily.
He was more relaxed. He wasn't in nearly as much pain. He
could smile again. A great improvement in the quality of his life.

I was able to see this patient for only three days before I
returned to the States. However, in that time, he learned that his
thoughts, and especially his responses to thoughts, could be
devastating to his health. He had witnessed and felt physical
changes brought about by his personal thoughts. And, once again,
I witnessed the powerful effects that emotions and thoughts —
current and past — can have on the body.

The patient and I talked at length about making correct
choices in thoughts and the rest of the six essentials. The
"Thought" essential deals with personal choices.

The patient himself took corrective measures. I didn't counsel
him — I'm not a counselor. My treatments weren't psychiatric
sessions — I'm not a psychiatrist. I helped him update the
inappropriate signals that kept his body ready to fight. The
emotions and their physiological responses were his. I can't take
them out of his brain, massage them into more appropriate shape
and put them back. He had to do it all himself. He had to
understand that the experience that prompted the emotions that
kept his body in non-stop defense was providing him a lesson in
living. He hadn't learned the lesson after the disappointing
business experience was over, so the lesson in handling disappointment and frustration continued. When he realized this and
reflected on the events that had led to his current problem, he
reevaluated the situation to find a positive lesson. I have no idea
what that particular lesson was for him. However, I do know
from my years of clinical experience that there is no such thing
as a negative lesson.

WELLNESS PRINCIPLE: Illness *or health* may be
                      self-inflicted.

I haven't seen this man since that brief three-day encounter.
I don't know how he is doing now. I do know that when I last
saw him he was on the road to recovery. Whether or not he
continued on that road, I may never know. However, I suspect
that if he begins to slide back into his old way of responding to
life's challenges he will recognize the symptoms and redirect his
thinking. Of course, my hope is that he is back on the tennis
court, exercising and improving his game and outlook on life.

Could exercise have helped this patient? Not when I first saw
him. His doctors had told him to exercise to maintain the little
muscle tone he had. However, had he done that, his condition
would have worsened. His muscles were already exhausted.
Some of them were contracted constantly. Trying to stretch a
contracted muscle can cause damage. And since many of his
muscles had nearly reached the limit of their endurance, exercise
would have made them more tired.

Exercise could have hastened his progress to complete
invalidism. His heart might have benefitted, but his skeletal
muscles wouldn't. He could have ended up in bed full-time with
a stronger heart and ever-weakening skeletal muscles.

WELLNESS PRINCIPLE: Yellow override keeps the
                      body responding to past-due
                      notices.

Yellow override can be the cause behind an assortment of
physical problems. Yet pain and disability are very real. The
focus here is on improving health, not curing disease. The
healing sciences have developed many techniques for alleviating
pain and addressing disease. When you hurt, the first order of
business is to reduce the pain. It's hard to think about the cause
when the effect demands your full attention.

I am definitely not advocating that you try to handle physical problems by adopting a Pollyanna attitude of positive thinking. However, positive thinking probably won't hurt.

If you are ill, consult a competent health-care professional and follow his or her advice. Then as symptoms are under control and you are able to look more positively toward the future, look at your health situation from a whole-body, whole-life perspective. That's what this book, and my other books, are designed to help you with — whole-body and whole-life health.

SPINDLES, ORGANS, AND ENGRAMS

The Red, Green, and Yellow are the "nerve centers" that direct movement and responses. But they need feedback information from the rest of the body to coordinate the movements and responses. We might say that the body is one big information loop. The central nervous system is in constant contact with physical structures throughout the body to coordinate whole-body functions.

For example, how do you keep from falling on your face when you stand and your body is balanced precariously on its rather narrow footing? How can you maintain your balancing act when you are walking or running? When you put your foot out to take a step, how does your leg know how far to go or when to stop?

It all happens below the level of consciousness. The cerebellum, located near the base of the skull, is in constant communication with the many muscles of the body. Your marvelous muscle machine is balanced and coordinated by an intricate information highway that links the brain, particularly the cerebellum, with sensitive feedback systems that report on current movements and performance throughout your musculoskeletal system. Your sense of balance begins with delicate equilibrium centers in your inner ear located within a few centimeters of the cerebellum. Information can be sent from inner ear to cerebellum in no more than a millisecond.[6] In contrast, information from feet to brain dawdles along at 15 to 20 milliseconds. Your feet can travel up to ten inches during that time lag.

Feet-information doesn't depend on your inner ear. Nor does hand-information. Movement of these outlying parts of your body are coordinated by information travelling between cerebellum and the muscles themselves.

We know that muscles are made up of tiny fibers. Skeletal muscle fibers contain tiny sensory receptors called muscle spindles. One job of muscle spindles is to serve as the keeper of muscle tone.[7] They send signals to the nervous system about the length or the rate of change of muscles.[8] Muscle spindles are stimulated by stretching and contracting. When a muscle is stretched, signals are sent to the nervous system fast enough to travel the length of a football field in about a second. And since we aren't football field length, the signals arrive at nerve centers quickly enough to adjust muscle speed and distance to keep movement under control. This balancing act of muscles contributes to smooth movements. Without this control, you might ram your hand onto your dining room table when you reach for your fork.

WELLNESS PRINCIPLE: Muscles and nervous sys-
                      tem communication allow
                      smooth moves.

Another muscle control structure that plays an important part in movement is the Golgi tendon organ. Tendons connect muscle to bone. Golgi tendon organs are in constant two-way communication with your nervous system. They provide information to the Green about the amount of tension of the muscles to which they are connected. They respond to subconscious instructions and report back to higher authority on their status.

So what do muscle spindles and Golgi tendon organs have to do with exercise, health, and the non-conscious?

Although you have no conscious control of either muscle

spindles or Golgi tendon organs, their activity is essential to any intentional movement. They communicate with your Green subconscious central nervous system as the Green responds to conscious intent. Muscle spindles and Golgi tendon organs also respond to messages that originate with emotions.

What's the main difference between conscious-intent messages and emotional messages?

Length of time. Duration. Your aerobics class or workout may last about an hour. Emotional distress can last days, weeks, or years. Muscle spindles and Golgi tendon organs don't question whether the orders they are responding to are serving short-term conscious intent or long-term non-conscious emotional stress. They just do their job. They are the worker bees that keep muscles tense even when you think you are relaxed.

> WELLNESS PRINCIPLE: Being tense is more than a
> state of mind.

Muscles respond to intention. Intention is a goal. When the phone rings, the goal is to answer it, not to control specific muscles. You don't consciously direct your movements. There's no mental monologue, such as, "I'm going to extend my left arm, carefully wrap the fingers of my left hand around the handset, adjust the tone and tension of my muscles to lift about eight ounces, gauge the distance and direction needed for the receiver to find my left ear, then nestle the instrument gently but firmly against my left ear without whopping myself in the head." If you had to consciously choreograph all of those movements, your answering machine would click on or the caller would hang up before you completed the instructions. Instead, the phone rings; you answer it. It's a conscious decision carried out by non-conscious memory of learned movement. Your nervous system, in cooperation with muscle spindles and Golgi tendon organs, takes care of the details. Your hand doesn't overshoot its destination. Once you grasp the handset, your arm doesn't swing

wildly toward the ceiling, nor do you hit yourself in the head
with the handset. It's all controlled movement. Your subconscious keeps track of the speed and direction of movement and
tension of muscles through messages from and to muscle
spindles and Golgi tendon organs.

The pattern for these movements has been stored in non-
conscious memory engrams. Engrams are patterns of memory
designed for the purpose of skilled motor function to aid in
survival. They allow muscles to perform practiced movement
faster than they could if you had to think about the movement.
Cutting with scissors, playing a musical instrument skillfully,
riding a bike, and answering the phone can be seen as patterns of
movement set in motion by information stored as memory
engrams.

> WELLNESS PRINCIPLE: Muscle spindles, Golgi
> tendon organs, and mem-
> ory engrams are the origi-
> nal labor-saving devices.

While these physiological labor-saving devices are helpful
most of the time, sometimes they are activated by emotions
rather than by conscious intentions. Muscles respond whether the
stimuli come from conscious intentions to accomplish a movement or from emotions that spark defense.

Emotions can keep muscles on guard and ready to defend for
a long time. When the subconscious nervous systems respond to
emotions, muscles tense and stay tense. But the muscles don't
carry out any defensive action. A non-conscious response pattern
is established for particular muscles. The same muscles stay
primed for action. Since this is now a learned non-conscious
response, whenever that emotion is triggered by an experience or
thought, the same muscle response is the result. So whenever you
are upset, the same pattern follows. The result may be a headache
or backache or neck ache or some other ache. It isn't a muscle

problem, it's a programmed Yellow non-conscious response.

WELLNESS PRINCIPLE: Muscles respond; they don't
analyze.

Responses to emotions prompted by experiences are what memories are made of. The non-conscious responds to memories. Memories — especially memories embedded by strong emotions — can serve as a template or blueprint for current response patterns. Suppose you were extremely frightened by a big, snarling, snapping dog when you were a small child. You vaguely remember the incident as just one of many childhood experiences. However, now, as an adult, you are tense and uneasy around dogs. It's a non-conscious response imbedded in memory.

If non-conscious uses memory engrams of past physiological responses as a pattern for current responses, then memories can affect how your muscles and body are performing right now. Non-conscious responses can affect your overall health and they can affect overall muscle tone and tension which, in turn, can affect your ability to exercise.

WELLNESS PRINCIPLE: The conscious mind is the
"seat of learning"; non-
conscious is the "seat of
health."

CHAPTER 5

SHAPING UP

FIRST THINGS FIRST

Exercise has a lot to do with the shape you're in — literally and figuratively. Exercise affects muscles throughout your body. It affects muscles that give your body shape, and muscles that keep your physiology in shape. The muscles that give your body shape are the muscles you learn to consciously direct so you can walk, throw a ball, bend, or turn over in bed. Muscles that keep your physiology in shape are the muscles under subconscious direction that keep your heart pumping, blood flowing uphill against the pull of gravity, food churning through your digestive tract, and countless other internal activities. So getting, or staying, in shape has greater benefits than merely improving your appearance. It can help improve your overall health. But remember, being "in shape," or "fit," doesn't guarantee health. And trying to "shape up" a body that isn't healthy could be dangerous. *Check with your doctor before starting any exercise program!*

> WELLNESS PRINCIPLE: An exercise program should
> be a health-enhancer.

We know that occasionally athletes in tip-top shape have had severe or fatal reactions while exercising strenuously. It's not that they weren't used to vigorous activity. These are people for whom regular strenuous exercise is a way of life. If strenuous exercise can bring on unexpected physical or physiological repercussions for the fit and hearty, their experiences should serve as a lesson for the rest of us. Have a check up by a qualified health professional before you shift your physiology into overdrive with exercise.

WELLNESS PRINCIPLE: Check up before you shape
up.

We saw earlier that excess protein may leave your internal environment struggling to retain its natural slight alkalinity. Cells produce acid as they work. The harder they work, the more acid they produce. Exercise has an acidifying effect on your body. The type of acid produced by cells is easily eliminated. But if your internal environment is already acid from too much protein food, even easily eliminated acid could push your acid factor into the danger zone. If you regularly eat a lot of high-protein foods such as meat, poultry, and dairy products, give your body a generous supply of foods that provide alkalizing minerals before you launch an exercise campaign. Begin by adding more servings of vegetables and fruits to your meals for a couple of weeks. A synopsis of how to improve your diet is found in the "Food Essential" section of Chapter 2. And if that merely whets your appetite to know more about diet and health, the first book in this series, *An Apple a Day?* goes into greater detail.

THE PURPOSE OF EXERCISE
The overall purpose of exercise is to keep *all* of the muscles in the body flexible, strong, and responsive so they can do their assigned jobs effectively.

The first lifestyle change many people make when they want to "get fit" and lose a few pounds is to start to exercise more. However, contrary to the premise that if you exercise enough you can eat anything you want and be slim, trim, and healthy, we have seen that "fit" doesn't necessarily equal health. Furthermore, exercise isn't the be-all, end-all of weight control. It can help, but it isn't the whole solution. Exercise mixed liberally with a predominantly alkaline ash-producing diet can point you in the direction of maintaining or regaining health. And when you are healthy, you have a better chance of living a long, productive, satisfying life. Indeed, exercise is the only defense against aging — if one needs a defense against this natural process.

Given time, we all age. As we age, reflexes slow, strength diminishes, and endurance lags. Usually, these changes occur so slowly that we barely notice them. Well-planned, well-executed, health-enhancing exercise combined with mineral-replenishing nutrition and an up-beat, find-the-good attitude toward every experience we have is the recipe for enjoying life and health no matter how many decades we have been around.

Whether we are young, old, or in transition between the two, we all need exercise. Each of us needs exercise appropriate to our individual condition.

Exercise is more than body-sculpting or strain and pain. Exercise is muscular motion. It is the voluntary or involuntary movement of muscles. And muscles of some sort move as long as you are alive. Your heart muscles move to keep blood flowing. Muscles between your ribs move to bring in and expel air. Even your esophagus is a muscular canal; muscular contractions move swallowed food into your stomach. And you don't give any of these physiological processes a thought. Muscular activity is part of living.

We talk about moving arms, legs, neck, and other body parts. Yet bones don't move without muscles pulling on them. We can't swallow food without the help of muscles. We can't smile, stand, breathe, or accomplish any other physical action without muscles that can relax and contract (tighten) in response to signals from our various nervous systems.

WELLNESS PRINCIPLE: Muscles are your movers
                      and shakers.

In order for muscles to be effective, they need to be able to
contract and relax. If you are constantly tense and "tied up in
knots," muscles are contracted unnecessarily. That's not only
exhausting but it reduces the muscles' ability to stretch. Proper
exercise can help to improve muscle tone and elasticity.

Health-enhancing exercise also benefits your cells as well as
the muscles of your internal organs and the muscles that move
bones. Muscles and cells need more oxygen when you exercise
than they do when you move at a more leisurely pace. And to
supply this increased oxygen demand, the heart pumps faster and
stronger to send more oxygenated blood through your circulatory
system. Periods of steady exercise increase your breathing and
heart rate and enhance cardiovascular efficiency. Exercise such
as running and fast walking strengthens the cardiovascular
system by helping to keep the heart and blood vessels strong and
resilient.

WELLNESS PRINCIPLE: Vigorous whole-body
                      exercise refuels your
                      cells with oxygen.

However, exercise benefits more than heart, lungs, and
skeletal muscles. Bending your arm involves more than just
muscles. Whether the arm-bend is to move food to your mouth,
pick up a bag of groceries, or shoot a hoop, tendons and other
connective tissue get into the act. Tendons attach muscles to
bones and other parts. But muscles and tendons don't function
independently. Highly sophisticated internal communication
networks of your nervous systems coordinate even the tiniest
movement. Scratch your head, lift a piano, or run the Boston
marathon, and your internal information highway buzzes with
messages and signals. Your central nervous system and all your

"little" nervous systems — autonomic nervous system, sympathetic nervous system, parasympathetic nervous system — get into the act.

WELLNESS PRINCIPLE: Your body can't do
                     anything without
                     responding to itself.

Without clear lines of internal communication, movement can come to a halt. So any exercise program you choose should include coordinated, complementary movements that keep communication pathways free of static and your nervous systems and muscles in synch. The exercise doesn't necessarily need to be vigorous or strenuous — just rhythmical and coordinated. Exercise that integrates internal communication involves movements that coordinate all quadrants of the body. More about that later. For now, keep in mind that proper exercise aids neuromuscular (mind/body) communication.

To summarize the purposes and benefits of exercise, proper exercise can:

1. improve muscle tone and elasticity,
2. enhance cardiovascular efficiency, and
3. reintegrate neuromuscular (mind/body) communication.

Your body is a superbly designed mechanism. It works best when all of its parts are allowed to do what they were designed to do. Movement is one of its outstanding design features. We're not rocks or trees stuck in one place until an outside force tears us from our moorings. Like a piece of fine machinery, the body needs to be used to keep it in good working order. It needs to move. It also needs to be supplied with nutrients it needs. You get your energy from the food you eat.

Muscles are the body's greatest energy consumers. Much of the food-energy (calories) you consume is converted to energy your body can use. When you consume more food-energy than you burn, the body stores some that can be used later for energy. We call that fat. The rule of thumb for losing weight is to consume fewer food-energy calories than you use. But how do we know if we are doing that, other than by watching the scales?

Tables of the calorie cost of physical activities show up in many books and articles on exercise and fitness. These tables give you an idea of how many calories are used by an hours worth of a particular activity. For example, snowshoe walking reportedly burns 4.5 calories per hour per pound of body weight. With that bit of information you can calculate that if you weigh 140 pounds and trudge through snow on snowshoes for an hour you will use about 630 calories.[9]

So your body needs proper "food fuel" that can be converted into energy. Your body runs on energy. For maximum energy, both physiological and physical, your body needs the best fuel you can give it.

WELLNESS PRINCIPLE: Use it or loose it, but fuel it with the good stuff.

YOUR MAGNIFICENT MUSCLE MACHINE

Your body has over 400 to 650 muscles, depending upon who is counting. Muscles come in assorted sizes, strengths, and job specialities. *Skeletal muscle* moves bones so you can move; *cardiac muscle* forms your heart, and; *smooth muscle* is a part of many internal organs. Skeletal and cardiac muscles have similar internal organization. The internal organization of smooth muscle is different from the other two, but, in general, the chemical basis for contraction is the same for all.

Our focus here is on skeletal muscles — muscles connected to bone. Skeletal muscle is the largest tissue in the body and makes up about 40% of body weight.[10] Muscles can do only two things: contract and relax. That's it. Every movement you make is accomplished by specific muscles contracting or relaxing on cue.

Many skeletal muscles come in pairs. They act as levers and they move joints. The individual muscles of a pair are antagonistic to each other; one has the opposite action of the other. When one contracts, the other relaxes. Biceps and triceps of the upper arm are an example of an antagonistic pair. When the biceps contract and the triceps relax, the forearm flexes at the elbow. With this action you can engage in a variety of activities — lift your fork to your mouth, raise your arm to comb your hair, scratch your ear, and that sort of movement. Relax both biceps and triceps, and your arm straightens and falls to your side.

But there's more to bending your arm than just biceps and triceps. Most movement requires the combined action of several muscles. When your biceps contract, your forearm may rise, but without the cooperation of other muscles, your hand obeys the law of gravity and bends down at the wrist. Movement requires more than just "prime mover" muscles that act to directly bring about the desired movement. It takes opposing antagonistic muscles, and the cooperation of synergistic muscles as well as the stabilizing effects of fixation muscles. Muscles must work together for smooth and accurate movement, and particular muscles may play different roles depending on the movement. However, no matter what the purpose of movement or how many prime mover, antagonistic, synergistic, or fixation muscles are needed to carry it out, all of those muscles are either contracting or relaxing. So, whether you are doing pushups, bench presses, or jumping hurdles, your muscles aren't pushing, they are contracting and relaxing. Muscles pull; they can't push.

WELLNESS PRINCIPLE: You can push only when
                      your muscles pull.

Although muscles appear to be large, bulky units, they are made up of many muscle fibers — from a few hundred to many tens of thousands. The fibers run the length of the muscle. Each fiber is made up of several thousand smaller structures called

myofibrils which, in turn, have millions of tiny molecular
filaments called myosin and actin filaments. These tiny myosin
and actin filaments overlap and can slide together. They are the
mechanisms of muscle contractions.

Now, this may be a bit more than you wanted to know about
muscles, but there's a point to all of this. When the actin
filaments are pulled alongside the myosin filaments, the fiber
contracts. And contractions are what muscles are all about.
Without muscle contractions, we can't move.

Not all contractions shorten muscles. The myosin and actin
don't always slide together. Isometric contractions tense muscles
but don't shorten them. An example of isometric contractions is
when you tighten your quadriceps to stiffen your knee joint. For
the majority of people, standing upright doesn't take much
conscious thought. We can stand because muscles contract
without shortening to keep us from falling over. Unconscious
muscle contractions maintain posture.

Isotonic contractions shorten muscles and keep tension
constant. Isotonic contractions are needed to lift a weight. Pick
up a bag of cement and your biceps not only tense, they contract
— isotonic contraction.[11]

Running is a mixture of isometric and isotonic contractions.
When you run, isometric contractions keep your leg stiff when
your foot hits the ground, and isotonic contractions move your
leg for the next step.

But what stimulates the muscles to contract?

Electrical current.

Small electrical current causes calcium ions to be released
into fluid inside the muscle fiber. The calcium ions initiate the
chemical reactions of the contractile process. Muscle movement,
then, is a physio-electro-chemical event. The mechanical
structure of the muscle is set in motion by electrical impulses that
spark chemical reactions. Muscles are some of the chief energy
burners in the body. You don't even need to be working them for
muscles to burn energy. And remember the calcium that the body

sometimes needs to keep your internal environment slightly
alkaline if there's not enough sodium to do the job? This is one
place the body can get it. From muscles. In the survival game, the
ability to contract muscles isn't nearly as survival specific as the
ability to keep blood slightly alkaline.

> WELLNESS PRINCIPLE: Muscle contractions use
> and produce energy.

The whole process of muscle contraction is an intricate mesh
of physical structure, electrical impulses, and chemical reactions
working together. Our muscles and their integrated movement
that we take for granted (when they work well) are an example
that the body works as a whole, complete, integrated system. In
order to keep muscles strong, resilient, elastic, and healthy, the
whole body must be healthy. And keeping the whole body
healthy is an ongoing process. Nothing in your body is static.
Everything keeps changing. Everything in the body affects
everything else in the body. That's why properly executed
exercise is important to health as well as to strength and a sleek,
"fit" appearance.

MUSCLE MAINTENANCE

Although some of us appear more muscular than others, muscle
design is standard. Fiber size makes the difference. Muscle bulk
or delicacy is determined first by heredity, later by physical
activity.

Muscle is "built" when the diameter of the muscle fibers
increases. Daily forceful resistive or isometric activity increases
the size of muscle fibers. To classify as muscle-building-forceful,
the muscle must contract to 75% of its maximum tension.[12] The
diameter of the fibers increases as the quantities of the internal
components increase. Sometimes, enlarged muscle fibers can
split lengthwise and form new fibers.[13]

WELLNESS PRINCIPLE: Resistance exercises
                      (isometric) help to "build"
                      muscle.

Prolonged weak muscular activity can build endurance, but
doesn't have much effect on muscle size or strength. Sustained
weak activity increases blood capillaries and oxygen carriers for
increased muscle metabolism. You may not get stronger doing
slow, steady exercise, but, over time, you'll be able to do it
longer.

WELLNESS PRINCIPLE: Regular, non-strenuous
                      exercise can help build
                      endurance.

On the reverse side of the muscle-building coin is muscle
atrophy, or wasting. Unlike people, muscles that don't exercise
lose size. After as little as a month of disuse, a muscle may lose
as much as half its size.[14] One of the most familiar examples of
this is after an arm or leg that had been strong and well-used has
been immobilized in a cast that inhibits movement. When the
cast is removed, the arm or leg is noticeably smaller than it had
been. The muscles are smaller from disuse. However, exercise
and physical therapy usually bring the muscles back to original
size and strength — a quick example of rebuilding muscle fiber.
    Although we can increase muscle size and endurance through
exercise, as we get older we lose muscle without working at it.
We even lose it as we sleep.

WELLNESS PRINCIPLE: Just living burns calories.

As you lie quietly in bed, your muscles use energy. Every
pound of muscle uses from 50 to 60 calories every day. It takes
that much calorie energy for muscles to function. This calorie use
has been termed passive metabolism.

Somewhere in their third or fourth decade, adults start to lose muscle mass at the rate of about a pound of muscle mass every year. Small wonder, then, that we find that bags of groceries or fertilizer feel heavier as the years go by. Of course, one pound per year is hardly noticeable.

If you lose a pound of muscle mass a year over 10 years, does that mean that when you are 45 years old you will weigh ten pounds less than you did at 35? Probably not. We seem to gain weight as time goes on. Most of us battle the creeping fat syndrome over the years. But even if your weight stays pretty much the same over ten years, the pound-a-year muscle loss means that ten of those pounds that were muscle mass are now fat. Fat doesn't burn calories. So now you have ten pounds less of muscle mass to burn the calories you take in. At the lower estimate of 50 passive-metabolism-calories per pound per day, if you are eating the same as you always have, 500 of those calories each day must be used for exercise or will probably be stored as fat. We can see that there are weight-control advantages as well as strength, endurance, and flexibility advantages to retaining or rejuvenating muscle mass.

WELLNESS PRINCIPLE: Exercise can help to retain
                                           or rejuvenate muscle mass.

Well, isn't building muscle mass what running, aerobics classes, tennis, working out, and all the other forms of exercise programs are all about?

It depends on what you do and how you do it. Running is essentially a lower-body, cardiovascular exercise. Great legs and great circulatory system. Tennis is essentially a legs and upper body exercise. Working out with weight equipment is generally directed toward building strength of specific muscle sets.

To either retain or rejuvenate muscle mass, muscles need to be exercised through their full range of motion. We need at least moderate exercise or movement to keep joints flexible and muscles supple (if not strong). The best way to maintain mobility and physical strength and to maintain muscle mass is to give your muscles the opportunity to work to their full capacity through full range of motion exercise. Full range of motion exercise allows major muscles and their antagonists to alternately fully contract and fully extend. Walking generally doesn't fit the full range of motion category. However, walking with exaggerated stride and arm swing does. To the observer, full range of motion walking may look a bit peculiar, but it also gives your cardiovascular system a good workout, reintegrates your neuromuscular communication, and improves muscle tone. We'll go into the how-to particulars in a later chapter. First, let's look at what we mean by that catch phrase "muscle tone."

THE HARMONY OF MUSCLE TONE
Recall the first benefit/purpose of exercise: Improve muscle tone and elasticity. Sounds like something athletes, trainers, and the locker room crowd might bandy about. But what does "improve muscle tone and elasticity" really mean? Just what is muscle tone? And aren't muscles always elastic, or stretchable?

Muscle tone is a steady state of slight contraction. It's the ability of a muscle to resist the force of gravity for long periods without relaxing. Sound tiring? You do it all the time.

Your subconscious controls the tonicity of your muscles. This is another of the marvelous design features that comes with the body package. Muscle tone doesn't need to be monitored consciously to make sure it's appropriate to the occasion. The degree of muscle tone changes according to what you are doing. When you are relaxed, muscle tone should be minimal. When you exercise, muscle tone increases as needed. Recall the internal communications we talked about earlier — your body talking to itself. Muscle tone is one of the topics of "conversation." Internal signals keep your subconscious apprised of the strength of contraction or relaxation of particular muscles. You decide consciously where and how you want to move a part of your body; your subconscious signals muscles to contract or relax to accomplish your purpose. You don't give a thought to how the process is handled. This "just do it and don't bother me with the details" arrangement allows you to use your conscious mind for other more interesting activities, such as bungee jumping and exploring the latest concepts of astrophysics. While you concentrate on accomplishing a task, your subconscious handles the details of doing it.

> WELLNESS PRINCIPLE: Conscious movement
> focuses on results, not
> process.

Muscle tone also contributes to your social image of being alert and keen-minded — muscle tone keeps your mouth closed when you are relaxed. Your lower jaw, with bones and teeth just hanging there unsupported, is subject to the laws of gravity. Presumably, you don't continuously concentrate on keeping your mouth closed when it's not being used for important activities such as eating, talking, singing, whistling, coughing, or gasping for breath. It's muscle tone that keeps slight tension on the muscles to hold the lower jaw up when you are relaxed. It's an involuntary response — you don't even have to think about it.

Muscle tone also helps you to stand upright. For example, your body is standing in line waiting for the movie box office to open, but your thoughts have wandered to tomorrow and an important meeting. You are standing still, but you have a lot of body that is teetering above the rather narrow foundation of your feet. Muscle tone keeps you from falling over. Muscles tense and relax as needed to keep you balanced. If all of your muscles were completely relaxed, joints would flex (bend) and you'd crumple in a heap. That's what happens when someone faints while standing and just sinks to the floor. Skeletal muscle tone virtually disappears.

On the other hand, when you are excited, muscle tone is

stepped up. Jumping for joy or in fright is muscle tone in high gear. Muscle tone fluctuates according to what you are doing and thinking. Sleep, fatigue, and anesthetics can decrease muscle tone. Excitement, either mental or physical, increases it.

A little personal experiment can demonstrate how muscles "turn on and off" when you appear to be completely immobile. Stand relaxed with your heels close together, hands hanging loosely at your sides. Stay as still as you can. By paying careful attention, you can feel very slight involuntary movements in your legs. If you stay that way for ten or fifteen seconds, you will feel yourself swaying ever so slightly. That swaying motion keeps you from falling over. And it's all automatic. It's muscle tone in action. The tone of skeletal muscles adjusts constantly to keep you balanced — and you don't even have to think about it.

You have probably had a physical exam where the doctor taps the area below your knee cap and your leg extends forward. This is the famed "knee jerk" reaction. Of course, science has a more sophisticated terms for it: "phasic myotatic reflex," or more simply "stretch reflex." Call it knee jerk or stretch reflex, it's an indicator of muscle tone.

WELLNESS PRINCIPLE: Muscle tone is muscles in
action when you're not.

But suppose your muscle tone stays maxed out when you are relaxed?

Aha! Now we're into elasticity.

Elasticity of a muscle is similar to elasticity of an elastic band. Compress it or stretch it and, when the pressure is off, it goes back to its original shape. Elasticity is the quality of returning to original size and shape after compression or stretching.[15]

Elasticity is a very important attribute of muscles. Muscles constantly stretch and contract and you certainly want them to be able to "un-stretch" or "un-contract." You have probably experienced strong involuntary muscle contractions that don't "un-contract" — the "knotted" muscle of muscle cramp or spasm. At that particular time, the muscle has lots of tone but no elasticity. Muscle cramps or spasms are usually painful. They can sideline fit, well-conditioned football players and other athletes.

Elasticity is the quality that makes muscles useful and reusable. Muscles that stretch (relax) and stay stretched are flabby — they lack tone. Muscles that contract and stay contracted are not only inelastic, they are overly tense and spastic. They can become tired and painful.

Of the three purposes of exercise, increasing muscle tone and elasticity have the most obvious overt benefits. Good muscle tone and elasticity allow you to move easily and smoothly. Without these two qualities, your movement is limited and you stand a good chance of hurting. And if you hurt, you are less likely to move enough to reap the benefits of increased cardiovascular efficiency and neuromuscular reintegration that we talked about earlier.

Exercise is more than a muscle-builder. It affects your whole body. Metabolism increases. Acid is produced. Energy is expended. Even your attitude is affected. Exercise affects the energy level of the body. That's a very important concept. The bottom line of fitness, health, wealth, and happiness is the grand total of your energy level.

CHAPTER 6

YOU'RE A BUNDLE OF ENERGY

ENERGY GIVE AND TAKE

You are teeming with energy. Energy throbs in and around you. You may not be able to direct internal energy toward activities such as steer wrestling or clog dancing, but you are "alive" with energy. Your energy level plays a big part in your health, wealth, and happiness. And, as you will see, energy itself is a guiding force in your life.

We are energy beings. We use energy. We produce energy. We live in a vast pool of energy. Whether or not we are as "energetic" as we would like, we are "full of energy." Everything that goes on in your body involves energy. Energy can be converted from one form to another. As Kenneth Ford puts it: "Like a clever actor who can assume many guises, energy appears in a variety of forms, and can shift from one role to another."[16] Energy takes the form of heat, light, color, and sound. Ford goes on to say, "Because of this richness of form, energy appears in nearly every part of the description of nature and can make a good claim to be the most important single concept in science."

There is "energy of mass" and "energy of motion," or kinetic energy. Matter, which includes us and the things in our visible world, has energy of mass. Matter is made up of atoms. Molecules are two or more atoms joined together. That's where the word "molecule" came from — Latin meaning "little mass." A molecule of water (H_2O), for example, is made up of two hydrogen atoms and one oxygen atom. Everything is made of atoms.

Atoms have mass, even though a single atom can't be seen with the naked eye. Atoms attract each other if they are a slight distance apart. They repel each other if they are squeezed too closely together. When a lot of atoms are linked together in a pattern, we have "something" — a droplet of water, ice, a rock, a plant, a duck, a person. But atoms aren't rigid. They vibrate and jiggle. They may not move from their set spot, as in ice or rock, nonetheless, they vibrate.[17] And vibration is motion — energy. So, since you are a breathing, thinking, mass of atoms, even when you are sitting still, you are vibrating and jiggling.

Heat energy is an accumulation of kinetic, or motion, energy. You get and accumulate energy from the foods you eat. Much of the food you eat has used light energy from the sun directly or indirectly. You eat plants, you eat animals that ate plants, and you eat products made from plants. Unassuming plants use the sun's light energy to transform inorganic substances such as water, carbon dioxide, and mineral salts into organic substances such as sugars, fats, and amino acids.

Functioning systems use only about 25% of available food energy in the process of converting food elements into a form cells can use. Most of the energy from food becomes heat. In the body, the rate that heat is "liberated" is generally referred to as the metabolic rate.[18] The terms "high metabolic rate" or "low metabolic rate" refer to how fast a particular body converts food and chemical energy to heat through chemical reactions.

WELLNESS PRINCIPLE: We take in energy and we
                       use energy.

Over 95% of the energy used by the body comes from the

reaction of oxygen with different foods.[19] Eating and digesting food is a form of energy conversion. The energy we get from food in the form of calories is converted to energy our cells can use to function. That's what a Calorie is: a unit of heat liberation.

But conversion to heat isn't the only way energy is used. Your muscles use energy when they work. Just moving an arm, leg, eyelid, or other parts of your body requires muscles to work. Moving the body strenuously requires more work, increases metabolic rate, and generates more heat.[20]

So, you take in light-energy that plants converted to substances your body can use, then your body converts those substances back into energy in a form your body can use for running processes and organs, or just plain running and other forms of movement. We might say that your body is in the energy business: it receives and processes raw materials and produces an energy product for internal use (cells, organs, processes, and all that) and external use (walking, lifting, bending, stretching, and all that). From the original light-energy source, we get heat-energy and kinetic-energy.

> WELLNESS PRINCIPLE: You are a living energy
> converter.

When we exercise, we convert energy from one form to another. As illogical as it may seem, the more energy we use to exercise, the more energetic we seem to be. (Of course, you can overexercise your body to the point of exhaustion, but that's not our topic of the moment.)

When we talk about energy in the body, we need at least a nodding acquaintance with "the energy molecule" adenosine triphosphate, or as it's usually called, ATP. So, a brief introduction to ATP.

THE ENERGY MOLECULE
The energy molecule, adenosine triphosphate (ATP), is produced

in the cells. You have about 75 trillion cells. We might say that each of us is a walking, talking mass of cells.

Cells are complex organisms. We won't go into the life and times of cells in depth. For now, we're concerned with the "energy factories" of the cell called the mitochondria (my-ta-KON-dree-a). One cell can have several thousand mitochondria. They are the "powerhouses" of the cell supplying about 95% of the cell's energy supply. Mitochondria convert nutrients and oxygen into the molecule ATP. ATP is the fuel cells need to perform physiological functions. It provides energy for virtually all cellular function. One of the jobs of ATP is to supply the energy to break the bonds that hold together the atoms that make up molecules of various chemical compounds. When the bonds are broken, electrons of the atoms "spin off." These electrons are then available to "mingle" with other atoms to form other molecules.

ATP is important when you exercise. ATP supplies energy needed during muscle contraction. The energy for muscle contractions comes from your cells.

WELLNESS PRINCIPLE: Tiny cell parts energize big
                       (and little) muscles.

Cells need oxygen. Earlier we referred to the blood as being an oxygen transport system. Cells need oxygen to produce energy from glucose. Glucose comes from carbohydrates in foods, especially whole grains, vegetables, fruits, peas, beans, honey, and even refined sugar. Plants make carbohydrates by using the sun's energy to combine carbon dioxide and water.

When we eat plants, the body turns the carbohydrate in the plants into glucose that the cells can use to make ATP. When enough oxygen is available to the cell, tremendous amounts of energy are released to make ATP. However, when oxygen is not available, or is in short supply, cells can still produce small quantities of ATP for "a few minutes."[21] That process is called anaerobic glycolysis — making glucose without oxygen.

Cells need to "convert" energy into usable form in order to be able to function. The raw materials for cellular function are oxygen and converted sun energy. We get the "sun energy" when we eat plants or animals that ate plants. Without ample quantities of both oxygen and sun energy, cells can't function properly, or at all. And cells need to function to sustain life. That's a pretty important concept — especially when it's your life that's being sustained.

Health begins in your cells. Healthier cells mean a healthier you. And the healthier your cells, the more energy you have. The more energy you have, the better you can move and do things, and the better your body functions. That's why its important for your diet to provide the nutrients your cells need to function, and the minerals it needs to keep your internal environment a comfortable place for them to work. Being kind to your cells is also the purpose of making correct choices in all of the six essentials. When you make the best choices possible in the six essentials, you keep your cells healthy, your internal environment "clean," and energy-producing ATP flowing.

> WELLNESS PRINCIPLE: Health begins at the cellular
> level.

YOUR BODY "TALKS" TO ITSELF

When we talk about ATP and the energy to rearrange molecules, we're talking mainly about energy produced by chemical reactions. Your body also uses and produces electrical energy. That's how it communicates internally. Body parts don't act without instructions of some sort. Instructions are transmitted by electrical signals. Electrical energy is transmitted along nerve fibers throughout the central nervous system and body to send messages to and from the brain and organs, muscles, tendons, and all other tissue.

Electrical connections of your brain and central nervous

system have a "sending" side (axon) and a "receiving" side (dendrite in the brain or neuromuscular junction in muscles). The space between "sender" cell and "receiver" cell is called a synapse. This isn't what we would term a big space. It's, as one source puts it, "only a few hundred wavelengths of light wide."[22]

The sender/receiver space isn't empty; it contains extracellular fluid. Electrical impulses that travel down the sending side axon cause chemical neurotransmitters to be released into the synapse. The neurotransmitters "drift" across the gap, and the chemical excites electrical energy in the receiving cell. Electrical impulses are transported by chemical transmitters. So, many of your electrical connections are really electrochemical connections.

Now, considering that brain and internal communication systems are constantly active and that literally millions of electrical and electrochemical messages are being transmitted constantly, you can see why we are energy consumers and energy producers.

WELLNESS PRINCIPLE:　We have so much electrical activity, it's a wonder we don't glow in the dark.

What does all of this have to do with exercise?

Recall the third Purpose of Exercise — reintegrate neuromuscular (mind/body) communication. Reintegrating internal communication is equally as important to health and fitness as the other two purposes of exercise: improving muscle tone and elasticity, and enhancing cardiovascular efficiency. But the need to improve internal communication doesn't get much press.

Your brain is your body's "command central." It "talks" and "listens" to every area of your body. Most of this two-way conversation is "top secret." That is, it's all subconscious. Your conscious mind is completely unaware of the subconscious messages that send precise instructions to particular muscles on how to find that itch on your ear, or how to move your arm and fingers to scratch the itch. And you don't give any thought to stretching or contracting particular muscles at a particular speed and intensity in a particular sequence so you can turn over in bed. Even if you are concentrating on precise movements, such as learning to ride a bicycle or play the piano, you concentrate on the results of neuromuscular coordination, not the process.

> WELLNESS PRINCIPLE: Conscious movement is goal oriented, not process oriented.

In general, activity in the right hemisphere of the brain controls the left side of the body, and activity in the left hemisphere of the brain controls the right side of the body. So repetitive exercise is most effective when movement alternates between the right and left sides of both upper body and lower body. This is the best kind of exercise to help balance your internal communication systems.

Walking *properly* is ideal exercise for reintegrating internal communication. A brisk rhythmic stride with arms swinging comfortably at your sides does more than exercise muscles and stimulate your cardiovascular and respiratory systems. Synchronized swinging of the right-arm-left-leg followed by left-arm-right-leg mimics the pattern four-legged animals use to walk. It also is the pattern pre-toddlers use in the important natural developmental process of crawling. Since walking is much easier on full-grown knees than crawling, follow the lead of our four-legged friends. Even though you're upright, when you are out for your evening stroll, walk, or jog, make sure you coordinate your arms with your legs. That way you'll get the neuromuscular integrating benefits of crawling and give your nervous system a chance to balance internal communication systems and body rhythms. Retoning your body's natural rhythms is equally as important as toning your muscles.

WELLNESS PRINCIPLE: The body seeks balance and
                        rhythm in its internal func-
                        tions.

YOU'VE GOT RHYTHM

You may not be able to carry a tune or maintain a syncopated
beat, but you've got rhythm. Even more startling, you've been a
rhythmical being since your conception. That's right. From the
time you were only one fertilized cell — long before anyone
knew there would be a you — you have been pulsating rhythmically. You began your rhythmicity even before your heart took
form and began beating. You had been around for four weeks
before that happened.

However, your heart isn't your only rhythm maker. Rhythmic
peristaltic action of smooth muscle of the intestines sends food
through your digestive system. Repetitive discharges of central
nervous system neurons keep your breathing rhythmical.[23] Even
the "proper" walking we talked about earlier is rhythmical. When
we talk about "the rhythm of life," it is more than just a poetic
phrase.

Not only do we have rhythm, we live in a rhythmical world
and universe. Days and nights, seasons, tides, movement of
planets all march to their own beat. But some of the rhythms are
so slow they are hard to detect.

Your body has its own rhythms. Within the greater rhythm of
birth, growth, and death are circadian rhythms — biological
activities that recur about every 24 hours — and a variety of
rhythms of renewal.

Your body maintains itself on cyclical replacement schedules
— out with the old, in with the new. Cells are lost and renewed
constantly. Cells of stomach lining are replaced in about five
minutes; the rest of the stomach takes about four days. Skin cells
are renewed monthly. Even the cells of our rock-solid framework
of bones are renewed in about three months. The atoms that make
up our component parts are ever moving. As Deepak Chopra

wrote in his book *Quantum Healing*, "Ninety-eight percent of the atoms in your body were not there a year ago."[24]

WELLNESS PRINCIPLE: You are a mass of dynamic
atoms.

The pulsating of a newly fertilized egg with no circulatory or cardiac system doesn't go away. Rhythmic pulses are a built-in feature of the body. One researcher identified four specific pulsations,[25] the first two being the most obvious and well-known:
1. A pulsation which is synchronous with cardiac contractions, and
2. A pulsation which coincides with respiratory pressure changes associated with inhalation and exhalation.

The third and fourth pulsations aren't as apparent:
3. A wave not related to either heart rate or respiration but one which constantly maintains its own cycle, and
4. An undulating pulsation which has not been identified.

What does rhythm, reconstruction, and restoration have to do with health and/or exercise?

A couple of things.

For one, it serves to emphasize that we pulsate with energy. We are creatures of rhythm.

We express rhythm in many physical activities. A smooth gait is rhythmic motion. And there's rhythm in nearly all sports, although the rhythm isn't always obvious. Ice skating, track and field, gymnastics, swimming, tennis, horseback riding, basketball, boxing, and even weight lifting capitalize on performing rhythmically. Less apparent is the rhythmicity of a forward pass or a throw from deep center field to second base, but it's there. Sports superstars make the most of their built-in rhythmic nature.

WELLNESS PRINCIPLE: "Poetry in motion" is more
than a metaphor.

The rhythm principle also demonstrates that both our lives and our bodies dance to beats. Rhythmic electrical energy is an integral part of our internal functions. Tiny electrical impulses travel along nerve fibers of the complex network of the nervous system.

Some internal energy-generating activities produce rhythms that can be recorded. Electrocardiograms (ECGs) are records of variations in electrical activity of the heart. Electroencephalograms (EEGs) are records of electrical rhythm and wave activity of the brain — alpha, beta, theta. ECG and EEG records are helpful diagnostic tools for assessing heart or brain function. But ECG and EEG records also indicate that electrical impulses can be detected on the surface of the body. Electrical energy "radiates" from your body.

WELLNESS PRINCIPLE: Your body uses and "gives off" energy.

However, the heart and brain are just two of the physical entities that produce energy. Everything made of atoms, molecules, and their subsections are members of the energy community. And since that includes all tangibles and many intangibles, we are relatively safe in saying that everything is energy.

Not too many years ago, students learned that the atom was the smallest, indivisible part of matter. That's what "atom" means in Greek: indivisible. However, as science and technology advanced, ever smaller subatomic parts have been discovered. Scientists have been able to identify smaller and smaller bits of matter until the matter is so small that it becomes pure energy. Einstein showed that very small amounts of matter have very large amounts of energy.

Atoms have a nucleus, which contains protons, neutrons, and at least one negatively charged electron circling the nucleus. Electrons spin as they circle the nucleus. Mobile electrons can spin off one atom and attach to another. This action binds the atoms together to make a molecule.

Researchers have "observed" electrons acting simultaneously as particles and waves. Since every atom has one or more electron, and since electrons are active, we might say that everything under the sun (as well as the sun itself) is in constant motion. Furthermore, moving electrons produce electromagnetic fields.

Whether we are consciously aware of it or not, energy is in and around us. We can't see, taste, hear, feel, or smell it, but it's there. We live in electromagnetic fields of energy generated by particles and systems that range in size from incomprehensively subatomic-tiny to incomprehensibly universe-large. These fields touch, overlap, interlace, and combine. Their energies pulsate with waves of rhythm. Whether you are meditating in a yoga pose or straining muscle, sinew, and nerve to complete a 26-mile marathon, you are functioning in an energy blender. And your body works best when your personal energy body is "in tune" with the energies that surround it.

WELLNESS PRINCIPLE: Harmony begins in your
home field.

ROMPING THROUGH THE FIELDS

Everything made of atoms and molecules is, and has, a field of energy. Animals, trees, rocks, birds, poison ivy, dogs, you, your neighbor — the entire earth. Your "personal field" is the ever changing total of the zillion electron fields that are included in (or are) your body. Your personal field is as much a part of your body as are your arms, legs, liver, teeth, and toenails.

We generally consider ourselves to be individuals roaming around on this planet. But when you look at yourself as an energy being, you see that you are an energy being with your own "external" energy field mixed in a universal cauldron with other fields. Your personal field abuts, bumps into, and intermingles with other energy fields. Consequently, you and your field can be

affected by and can affect other energy fields. Your field alone
isn't all that big — several inches around your body. But your
field constantly contacts other fields. Your energy mixes with the
energy of fields around you which in turn affect other contiguous
fields. An instantaneous reaction of "He-really-turns-me-off" you
may have to an individual may be more of a field response than
malice.

Your field constantly blends with fields around you. It's
rather like the dash of salt you put into chicken soup. Once the
salt goes into the mixture, it affects the whole brew. So we might
say that we live in a cauldron of energy soup. Since fields
overlap and intermingle, your personal field is a part of this
energy soup. And your personal field is your direct connection to
the universal field.

> WELLNESS PRINCIPLE: Just by being, you affect the
> world and the world affects
> you.

The energy of the field of each of us is perfect. However,
some personal fields are less vibrant than others. The personal
field "ebbs and flows" depending on the amount of interference
from without or within. So although fields are fields, their
intensity and vibrancy can change according to the interference
that is affecting the field at the moment. We might think of
interference as being like static that muddles the reception of
radio signals, or "snow" that obscures the picture on a TV. The
signals are being transmitted and received, but they can't get
through loud and clear. Where does this static that interferes with
our field communication come from?

All around us.

In our high-tech society, we live in close proximity to many
man made electrical and electronic systems. "Leakage" of energy
from these systems can affect your field. And, your field can be
affected by interference from inside your body. Food, and

anything else that enters your body, can affect your field either positively or negatively. Thoughts, memories, and emotions can affect your field either positively or negatively. Negative thoughts, memories, and emotions are generally high intensity energy conductors that can "pollute" your field and reduce its vibrancy.

When static interferes with clear transmission of energy between fields closely connected to your body, communication within your body can suffer. Internal rhythms can be "desynchronized," and internal communication can be disrupted. And the big problem with interference is that it jumbles the communication flow of your personal field that connects you with the Perfect Intelligence of the universe. If there is interference in your field, there is interference in your energy connection with the Ultimate Source of Power. And when your energy connection is less than top notch, your internal energy level and flow suffer.

WELLNESS PRINCIPLE: Your personal field is your
conduit to Perfect Universal
Intelligence.

Magnetic and electromagnetic fields are produced by electrical current. Electron activity produces electrical currents and electromagnetic fields. Electrons carry a charge, and they carry "information." The "information" carried by each electron is identical; only the vehicles vary.

An electron is an electron. There aren't people electrons, liver electrons, brick electrons, tree electrons, fly eye electrons, and the like. Electrons retain their characteristics. It's atoms that change as they gain or lose electrons. A fly-eye electron can serve equally as well as a stainless steel electron, a computer chip electron, or a passion fruit electron. The reason electrons are so versatile is that they all carry the same "information." This "information" is the Perfect Intelligence, or Universal Energy, that runs the universe and everything in it.

Perfect Intelligence information isn't the same as knowledge, such as understanding the concept of $2 + 2 = 4$. Perfect Intelligence is the Ultimate Power Source of everything necessary to run the universe and all of its parts. As far as your body and health are concerned, Perfect Intelligence is the power behind your systematic development from one fertilized egg to an integrated system of 75 trillion (give or take a few billion) cells.

When you were the original one-cell that evolved into you, all of the intelligence needed to turn you into a complete person was present in and around that one cell. You were not only one cell, you were one cell equipped with your own personal field of information.

But, how could your field be yours personally when you were inside your mother and her field?

Your field became personal as soon as the sperm and its field joined with the egg and its field. Instant individual field.

A fertilized egg cell begins as a "two-piece package" — fertilized egg and field. Development begins when the egg begins to duplicate its genes then divides into two identical and complete cells in a process called mitosis. These two cells then divide, or reproduce themselves to become four identical cells. Then the four become eight cells, the eight become sixteen, and so forth. But it takes more than continuous replication of identical cells to produce a fully-formed small person. So, at the proper time, cells begin to differentiate. Some become nerve cells, some blood cells, some tissue cells, some muscle cells, and some every other type of cell needed to complete the package.

Now the question is: how do cells "know" how and when to differentiate to become cells for particular organs and structures? How does a cell know how and when to become a heart cell, or pancreas cell, bone cell, or whatever? And how do these cells know where to form a particular part of the body? There's no brain or nervous system to direct the operation. And the mother isn't the construction boss. As one physiology textbook puts it: "In the normal human body, regulation of cell growth and reproduction is mainly a mystery."[26] The electrochemical component or activity hasn't yet been "scientifically" validated. Nonetheless, Chopra, who views the body as being greater than tissue, fluids, and electrochemical reactions calls the intelligence we're talking about "know how."[27] In the body, the intelligence responsible for regulating growth and development is Perfect Intelligence "know how." The body, through its energy connection with Perfect Intelligence, has the "know how" to differentiate cells to develop organs where they will have the best protection, such as hiding the heart, lungs, and other vital organs in a bony rib cage, and protecting the delicate brain with a thick skull.

WELLNESS PRINCIPLE: Our configuration, as well as our response systems, was designed for survival.

We develop as a whole, not piece by piece. Development follows an intricate plan. The design and construction plan is more complex and comprehensive than anything Generic Man has devised, or, more likely, can devise. Generic Man doesn't grow a computer, a suspension bridge, or a space vehicle. These are built piece by piece. The blueprints for them show the finished product, but the pieces must be constructed and put together. Not so with the body or other living entities. Living structures aren't put together; they emerge.

From the beginning of the development process, the ultimate product is defined by its field. This phenomenon was demonstrated in the 1920s by Harold S. Burr, a neuroanatomist at Yale University. Burr found that the field around a developing seedling was in the shape of the adult plant; not in the shape of the original seed. The field appeared to be a template, or pattern, for growth. The plants grew into their fields. We seem to do the same thing. We can assume that the field that surrounded our single fertilized egg was the template for our finished product body and is the same field we live in our whole lives.

> WELLNESS PRINCIPLE: We grow and develop in, and into, our own field.

Your personal energy field is not only with you all the time, it is a permanent part of you. It is as much a part of you as your skin. As long as you live, your field is your connection with all of the Ultimate Power Source intelligence your body needs to function at its best. My clinical experience and research indicate that the ill-health of many patients may be connected to interference in the patients' personal energy fields. We could say that we are energy beings experiencing a physical existence.

We might go so far as to say that health hinges on energy mingling freely through body and field. When interference of any kind impedes the natural energy flow, we may experience discomfort or agitation of some sort.

With the growing amount of man-made electrical devices and systems of our high-tech society, our individual fields are bound to be affected by external interference. However, external interference is only one source of interference. Internal interference brought on by physical, emotional, and nutritional stress can have an impact on the health and vitality of our personal fields. Individually, we may not be able to control external conditions, but we can control our choices of the six essentials to reduce the amount of field interference that originates internally.

We are energy beings. We are energy; we consume energy; we radiate energy, and; we live in a universally-connected energy environment. Health is energy sensitive. When transmission of energy information in or between the many interconnected energy fields is impeded or interfered with, your health (the way your body functions) may be affected. The choices you make in the six essentials can help to promote your energy level. And we have seen that there's more to your energy level than just how energetic you feel. In previous chapters, we touched on how nutrition and thought choices can interfere with health. Now let's take a closer look at how exercise fits into your physical and field health.

CHAPTER 7

STRESSING EXERCISE

STRESS REVISITED

We have talked about muscles, motion, tone, mass, contraction, relaxation, and the energy components of the body. Now it's time to relate these elements to the concept of the whole body condition. Stress, no matter what its source, is certainly a whole-body condition.

Earlier on, we defined stress as any stimulus that changes the way the body is functioning. With that understanding, we can see that every time a muscle moves, conditions change internally. Muscles use oxygen. The oxygen must be replaced. Muscle activity produces acid. The acid must be eliminated. Every movement — conscious or subconscious — alters internal conditions and the body must respond. Stress.

Yet, the biggest internal stimulators of all come from thoughts and emotions that originate in the brain. Mental and emotional activity has a greater effect on the body and health than exercise, diet, breathing, and rest put together. Your brain is constantly active. The Green functions even when Red and Yellow activity is at a minimum. And what does the brain control? In addition to being the seat of thoughts, emotions, and "the mind," the brain controls every internal function and physical activity. So your physical brain (which can be seen and explored) and your mind (which has yet to be adequately defined) are the ultimate stress producers.

WELLNESS PRINCIPLE: Stress is an inside job.

The body is designed to handle stress. It's part of the survival process so you can fight or run away from a threatening tiger. Problems crop up when your body must respond to the same "tiger" stress for long periods. Year after year of living in a war zone is repetitive "tiger" stress. Physical danger is present over and over — the "tiger" keeps charging. But for most of us in this country, long-term stress doesn't come from the outside world. It is self-generated.

"Oh-ho," you say, "you don't have my job. Too much to do, too little time to do it, and people crawling on my back. That's stress."

Okay, let's look at job stress.

Whether you work for yourself, your family, or someone else, every job comes with pressures. Tasks must be accomplished within a given time. Personalities must be accommodated. Mistakes must be held to a minimum. A job may be pressure-packed, but "job stress" usually isn't the result of physical threats. Job stress is a mental response. Worry, fear, guilt, anger, anxiety, and frustration are mental responses that spark internal physiological responses. Organs, systems, and muscles adjust to consciously perceived threats. The result is defense; survival physiology. We respond physically and physiologically to stimuli that we consciously interpret as threats. It's the old "stick-snake" syndrome. If you "see" a snake as a stick, the object is non-threatening. The perception is but a tiny blip in your consciousness. If you "see" it as a snake, no matter what the object is, you and your physiology respond. The sympathetic side of your autonomic nervous system takes charge immediately. You're primed for action!

WELLNESS PRINCIPLE: For your body, thinking
                      makes it so.

As far as your body and physiology are concerned, being
primed for action to get away from or kill a snake is no different
from being primed for action to defend against job stress. Your
sympathetic nervous system is in charge of preparing for fight or
flight. When your Red intellect detects a threat, your Green
subconscious responds with sympathetic survival adjustments.
Your Green doesn't analyze the situation to determine if the
threat is one that will wound your body or merely wound your
ego. It doesn't differentiate between an immediate physical threat
posed by a knife-wielding mugger and an intangible threat of a
potential financial disaster posed by a notice that your employer
is downsizing. When your Red picks up a threat, your Green
responds for survival —   heart pumps harder, blood is
concentrated in muscles, heart, and brain, organ functions slows.
Adrenaline rush. Survival response.

WELLNESS PRINCIPLE: Stress isn't what happens to
                      you; it's how you respond to
                      what happens to you.

Occasionally, we need a quick survival response to avoid a
real physical threat. However, we don't need to inflict non-stop
survival responses on our bodies when we're not in physical
danger. Of course, if your house is blown away by a tornado,
that's stress — even if you're not in it at the time. Personal
catastrophes are legitimate stress. Yet after the initial shock and
trauma are over, your body is designed to get back to
maintenance-repair balance.

I'm not suggesting that you try to turn off all emotions in
order to keep stress responses under control. For one thing, you
can't "turn off" emotions. You can merely repress them — tuck
them away where they don't bother you consciously. As Henry

David Thoreau said over a hundred years ago: "The mass of men lead lives of quiet desperation." Emotions are always with us. They need to be expressed — in a civilized way. The expression can be as subtle as a smile or frown. Perhaps a hearty laugh, a "good cry," an impromptu little dance of delight, a sharp-tongued comment, a scathing letter to the editor, or a sweat-generating physical workout. But violence and bloodshed are out. Emotions, particularly strong negative emotions, that are kept bottled up can eventually be expressed by the body as chronic illness, pain, or catastrophic ill-health. Until emotions are expressed in some way or another, they can sit below consciousness, prompting defense responses, and possibly setting the stage for future discomforts.

What about all of the emotions from negative experiences you managed to suppress in the past? Very likely they are still affecting your physiology — Yellow override. The experiences, along with the physiology they generated, are stored in memory. Tight or flaccid muscles, subdued or non-stop digestion, high or low blood pressure can be ongoing responses to stimuli stored in memory. But you aren't doomed by your past. When a thought of a past unpleasant experience flits through your mind, you can recognize it as a stored-stress situation that put you in defense. Think about it and find some element of good that will generate a germ of satisfaction or pleasure. Then dwell on the positive element. This process can be especially effective when used in conjunction with the "Morter March" which will be explained later. You will find that after satisfactorily completing this exercise a few times, the thought recurs less and less frequently. But if it does, focus on the positive element you found in the experience.

This thought-exercise may sound like a bit of whimsy. However, it can be quite effective in reducing residual stress. And it's residual stress that is behind most of the physical ills that are so prevalent in our society today.

WELLNESS PRINCIPLE: Emotions will be expressed

sooner or later.

ADRENALINE — FRIGHT OR EXCITE

Many people seem to live their lives on an emotional roller coaster. Sometimes it's a baby coaster with rolling hills and hollows that rarely deviate from level. Other times it's like the "Texas Giant" super coaster with its succession of highs and lows, thrills and chills. There's a fine line of distinction between terror and thrill — one person's thrill is another person's terror. Yet from your body's perspective, whether it's terror, thrill, or ecstasy, excitement is excitement. The excitement of watching your favorite team in a close contest can affect your body in a manner similar to the excitement of fear and rage. Adrenaline rush.

Adrenaline (or epinephrine, as it is also known), is produced by the adrenal glands. The standard body model comes with two adrenal glands; one gland atop each kidney. And as a bit of trivia to mesmerize your friends, "adrenal" gets its name from "kidney"; it's from Latin *ad*, meaning "to," and *ren*, meaning "kidney." Adrenal glands secrete a variety of very important hormones.

Hormones are chemical substances. They are secreted by a cell or group of cells and have a controlling effect on the activity level of other cells. Hormones come in many varieties. For most teenagers, and parents of teenagers, the word "hormones" implies sex hormones. While ovarian and testicular hormones can turn cute kids into turbulent teens, many other hormones play vital but less conspicuous roles. Pituitary hormones, thyroid and parathyroid hormones, pancreatic hormones, and other hormones with tongue-twisting names are concerned with controlling metabolic function.[28]

Adrenal glands secrete two different types of hormones. The adrenals are like two glands in one. The outer layer of the gland — the adrenal cortex — secretes mineralcortocoids that affect the electrolytes of extracellular fluid, and glucocorticoids that affect

carbohydrate, protein, and fat metabolism. The inner portion of
the gland — the adrenal medulla — secretes epinephrine
(adrenaline) and norepinephrine.[29] These are the hormones that
give you that adrenaline high when you are overly excited or
"pumped up."

And another bit of trivia that won't change your life, but you
may find interesting: Recall that earlier I talked about how we
develop as a whole from one cell — not as a ready-for-assembly
package of parts. The adrenal glands get their dual-function
ability from the way they develop. The outer layer cortex
develops from the same embryonic tissue as the reproductive
glands. The inner, or medulla, portion develops from the same
embryonic tissue as the sympathetic nervous system.[30] Hence, the
close relationship between the outer layer and adolescence, and
the inner portion and fight-or-flight.

Adrenaline production is part of the body-wide network of the
fight or flight response stimulated by your sympathetic nervous
system. The conscious mind detects a threat and the subconscious
sympathetic system responds — ready for battle. The
sympathetic system alerts the whole body via nerve pathways.
Included in the body-wide alert are signals that race along nerves
to cells of the adrenal medulla that secrete adrenaline and
norepinephrine (also called noradrenaline).

Adrenaline is potent stuff. It can increase the metabolic rate
of the body as much as 100%, which increases the activity and
excitability of the whole body.[31]

WELLNESS PRINCIPLE: Adrenaline is the "booster
                      rocket" for survival
                      responses.

The excitatory effect of adrenaline isn't a big secret. So,
what's the big deal?

The body was designed to produce adrenaline in direct
response to an immediately threatening physical encounter.

Signals from any of the five senses alert the whole body through the autonomic nervous system of immediate danger to life and limb. The big deal about adrenaline is that man has learned to stimulate its production with his mind when no actual physical danger exists. Both fear of the future and fear of a charging tiger cue adrenaline production.

Adrenaline has much the same effect on the body as the sympathetic nervous system. But its effects are more far-reaching. Adrenaline can affect the metabolic rate of *every* cell of the body. Although the sympathetic system can control body-wide functions such as arterial pressure or metabolic rate, the nerve connections of the sympathetic system directly affect only a small portion of cells of the body.[32] And since adrenaline and norepinephrine are delivered into the blood, adrenaline effects last five to ten times as long — up to a minute or two — as sympathetic nerve stimulation.[33] When you become excited in your conscious mind, your subconscious activates sympathetic and parasympathetic responses and epinephrine and norepinephrine flood your body. The result is defense physiology.

For example, there you are at your trusty work station chaffing under the pressures of the job. What's happening in your body? Your sympathetic system is responding to a job stress "threat" and adrenaline is coursing through your body. But you don't run. You don't fight. And the adrenaline with its residual effects keeps coming. Your internal systems stay on guard. Your body is in a constant state of sympathetic tone. Tense. Ready to fight. Sympathetic dominance. What's a body to do?

Well, unless you do something to "burn off" the adrenaline, your body will stay uptight. You could scream, rant and rave, and jump up and down. You could put your fist through the wall. You could have a temper tantrum. But none of those responses is socially acceptable. So what do many of us do? We grit our teeth, clench our fists, knot our stomachs, or tense our muscles and go on. We go on with our bodies working faster and harder. But we don't "work off" the adrenaline. Then, at the end of the day, we wonder why we are tired when we haven't done much in the way of physical exercise. The common perplexity: How can sitting at a desk all day be so tiring? Now you know. It's not all imagination. The body has been working hard even though it hasn't moved around much. Adrenaline has been pumping. Defense mechanisms have been working at full tilt. But muscle movement was being restrained. That's why many people find that vigorous exercise after work is a tension reliever. It helps use some of the adrenaline that's been flooding the system all day.

If internal systems are constantly prepared for flight or defense, a civilized way must be found to uncork the pressure that is bottled-up by daily stressful frustrations. Exercise is a good corkscrew.

Now, this gem of wisdom is hardly a new concept. Many of us know intuitively or by experience that vigorous exercise acts as an antidote to frustration, anger, and anxiety. Now you can see why. These "ready to fight" emotions stimulate sympathetic responses and keep the adrenaline level high. And if the frustration, anger, and anxiety are constant, the adrenaline surge is constant. Exercise helps to put the adrenaline to good use and brings the body back into balance.

Exercise is good. But it isn't the last word in becoming healthy. Those who must run several miles a day to feel good are taking an "exercise aspirin." Running can be enjoyable and health-enhancing. But routinely running to get rid of excess adrenaline is treating symptoms. Different choices in attitude are called for to reduce the mind-generated adrenaline. As long as the same old choices in responding to daily situations are made, more and more exercise will be needed to get the same results. This year six mile runs. Next year, twelve mile runs may be needed to get the same effect. But pretty soon, some organ or system of the body wears out because the runner didn't address the cause.

WELLNESS PRINCIPLE: You shouldn't have to exercise to feel good.

Those who are in a constant state of worry, depression, and lethargy aren't generally inclined to hit the road for a good run. Worry, depression, and lethargy stimulate the parasympathetic response. As we noted earlier, *in general,* parasympathetic responses have a subduing effect on the body. And since worry, depression, and lethargy are usually long-term conditions, the parasympathetic system is continually stimulated. Muscle tone is reduced; gastrointestinal activity increases. Saliva production, pancreatic secretions, rectal and bladder activity all increase. Adrenaline production is at a low ebb. Parasympathetic dominance. Parasympathetic responses are designed for rest and repair. However, for the worrier, resting isn't restful. It's exhausting. Parasympathetic dominance leads to the curl-up-in-a-corner-and-suck-your-thumb response to life, and to under-toned muscles.

WELLNESS PRINCIPLE: Either sympathetic dominance or parasympathetic dominance is exhausting.

Does that imply that parasympathetic-excess worriers shouldn't exercise or that the sympathetic-excess, angry and frustrated should chuck their day jobs and train for the Olympics?

No, indeed!

Exercise can help those at either extreme of the autonomic response scale, as well as those with less obvious responses.

Keep in mind that every function of the body is aimed toward survival and that every survival response is perfect. The body can't do anything wrong. A continuous flood of adrenaline, excess muscle tone, meager muscle tone, sympathetic excess, or parasympathetic excess are all survival responses to particular choices in the six essential areas.

    WELLNESS PRINCIPLE: Life is an exercise in sur-
                                 viving stress.

SURVIVING STRESS

There's no getting around it: we have endless opportunities in life to practice handling tension and upheaval in our lives. To put it another way, life is a series of stress and trauma lessons. Lessons in making appropriate choices. We are given the opportunity to make choices throughout our lives. When we habitually make appropriate choices in each of the six essentials, our lives, physiology, and bodies have better opportunities to sail along on relatively smooth waters. When we make inappropriate choices, life can be turbulent and health can be impaired. And since life is one vast learning experience, the more inappropriate choices we make, the more opportunities we will have to repeat the lessons.

    WELLNESS PRINCIPLE: Stressful situations are life's
                                   classrooms.

    Some of us have trouble paying attention in our classes of life. We don't always recognize a lesson when it comes along. Perhaps you know someone who has been married and divorced two or three or four times. They are in a rut. Each of the spouses is virtually a carbon copy of the one before. This succession of fractured relationships provides a lesson to be learned. When you see life as a series of lessons, you can see that the frequent-marrier just isn't learning the lessons being presented. They keep repeating inappropriate choices, miss the point of their personal lessons, and wonder why their life is so tumultuous and their general health isn't as good as they would like.

    We begin learning lessons when we are children. With adequate social conditioning as children we learn to glide or stumble along with a minimum of stress through encounters and

relationships with others. But many of us don't grasp the need for
stress conditioning until we reach adulthood. That's when
symptoms of "hyperactive" sympathetic dominance or "lethar-
gic" parasympathetic excess usually become most apparent. Both
are responses to thoughts, and both can create timing problems.
We can see the need for sympathetic dominance to fend off
physical danger. But what about parasympathetic excess? How
does that fit into the survival picture?

The body seeks balance. It has a sympathetic excitatory mode
and a parasympathetic relaxation mode. Ideally, the sympathetic
and parasympathetic systems work in concert to keep your
internal energy and physiology in healthful, balanced homeostasis.

When the sympathetic system is in charge, you are alert and
ready to meet all manner of challenges. When your parasympathetic system is in charge, you are in your triple-R mode — rest,
repair, and refuel. Your body needs time and opportunity to take
care of these crucial functions.

We have seen that emotions of worry and depression can
stimulate parasympathetic responses. But worry and depression
aren't particularly relaxing. They are submissive rather than
aggressive emotions. Submission is a survival technique. No
need to flex muscles and leap tall buildings when you are
submitting. But continuous parasympathetic responses are as
hard on your body as are continuous sympathetic responses.
When parasympathetic responses dominate, the digestive system
churns even when there's no food to work on. Muscle tone
decreases. Adrenaline secretion is at low ebb.

Exercise can help you and your body bounce back if your
physiological responses are being controlled by inappropriately
timed parasympathetic dominance. Exercise stimulates the
muscular system. Activity of the muscular system stimulates the
sympathetic system which stimulates adrenaline production. So
when a parasympathetic-dominant person exercises, the sympathetic system rises to the occasion and the systems are brought

closer to balance. That's the secret to surviving stress: body balance. That's also the objective of learning to make appropriate choices in the six essentials. When appropriate choices in each of the six essentials far outweigh inappropriate choices, you are better able to reach your personal best in balance.

Life is one lesson after another. With each challenge, your job is to figure out what lesson problem you just solved. If you don't figure it out, you'll repeat it until you learn it.

Approach stressful situations with a positive attitude. Recognize that you have choices in your life and lifestyle. You have choices in how you conduct your life, and you have choices in how you respond to others. Recognize that you will make choices that you think are mistakes, and that you won't always make correct choices to meet the goals you have set for yourself. That indicates that you are still learning. Every once in a while, take a hard look at your lifestyle and don't be afraid to make changes.

WELLNESS PRINCIPLE: Stress and other symptoms
are choice opportunities.

STRESS CAN BE A PAIN

We are a time-oriented species. "Time is money," we're paid by the hour, and schedules control our lives. But time in months, weeks, days, hours, minutes, seconds, and nanoseconds is a conscious mind concept. The Green doesn't understand time. It doesn't know the difference between today, tomorrow, yesterday, or fifteen years ago. It responds to current internal stimuli. The Green doesn't care if stimuli are coming from a current event, the memory of a past event, or the anticipation of a future event.

We have talked about how Yellow-stored memories include both our interpretation of the "facts" of an experience and the pattern for the physiology that accompanied that experience — drill sergeant Uncle George and all that. Memory is much more than recollection of past events. Memory is also behind the personality characteristics we develop. We learn early on which behaviors make us feel good. Or, if not feel good, which behaviors cause us the least physical and emotional pain: aggressiveness or submission, perfectionism, ambition, competitiveness, conscientiousness, or indifference, self-acceptance, self-hate. Once we learn which behaviors are the least traumatizing, we follow those behavior patterns. And along with the behavior seen by the outside world are emotions that govern internal worlds.

We try to avert as much mental anguish as possible. But we aren't always successful. We slip up. We forget appointments — so much for conscientiousness. A project falls short of perfection. A relationship turns sour. So what do we do?

Not much physically. As mature adults, we don't scream and holler, and jump up and down. But the Green can tell muscles to be ready for action. So tighten up muscles. Contract. And until the Green releases them, those muscles will stay contracted. Even if we consciously try to relax, some residual contraction remains. But this isn't the first instance of unresolved contraction. If you are carrying around overly contracted muscles from Uncle George and incident after incident is piled onto this response, eventually you not only have tight muscles, you may have pain. It might be back pain, shoulder pain, headache, elbow pain, or sciatic (leg) pain. The same pain response can come from one big, catastrophic incident. Responses to a series of small incidents or to one humongous incident can bring on a severe contraction we call spasm. And muscle spasms hurt.

WELLNESS PRINCIPLE: Subconscious responses can
cause pain.

We know intuitively that pain is the body's signal that something isn't quite right. Muscle pain signals are loud and clear. However, muscle pain brought on by emotional upheaval can be more than a physical response of muscles — it can be a physiological response. An emotionally-induced muscle spasm can hurt just as much as a physical injury from a weekend touch football escapade. Yet a physiological response is different from a structural or physical injury. The difference is in the condition of the muscle. A muscle that is painful as a result of emotions is as healthy as it was before it went into spasm. The muscle doesn't have a problem. Inappropriate internal messages are prompting perfect, but ill-timed, responses. The body never does anything wrong. It responds perfectly to every stimulus or message.

Of course, the source of severe muscle pain — or any pain — should be determined by a health care professional. If the doctor finds that the problem isn't structural and finds no physical cause, your body may be responding to emotions.

When physical pain grabs your attention, emotional pain can recede from consciousness. It isn't eliminated; it's just pushed into the background. Recognizing that pain can come from emotional responses is the first step in recovery from emotionally-induced pain.

WELLNESS PRINCIPLE: Muscle pain distracts from
emotional pain.

We often treat pain, especially stress-induced pain, by taking pain-relievers. That treats the symptom, but does nothing to get at the cause of the pain. It's a temporary solution. And that's fine to help you get through the work day, or to get to work at all. If every worker with a stress-induced headache or backache stayed home, the stress on our personal and national economies would be overwhelming. Taking pain-relievers can help minimize work loss. Just recognize that it is a "band-aid" solution. It's like taking antihistamine to "dry up" a runny nose. It takes care of the immediate symptom, but doesn't "cure" anything. Ignoring the underlying cause — poor choices in the six essentials — assures that the same or more severe symptoms will show up later. Remember: The body can't do anything wrong. Pain is your body's way of telling you that something needs to be changed.

WELLNESS PRINCIPLE: Pain may be a symptom of
                      poor choices.

When we hurt physically we tend to limit our activity. That's a natural inclination. But stress-induced pain doesn't benefit from pampering. That just focuses on the pain. Moderate exercise can help relieve stress-induced pain. It improves neuromuscular timing, works off adrenaline, and improves oxygen-carrying blood flow to muscles.

A full-complement of blood supply to muscles is important for both you and the muscle. A "well-fed" muscle is a "happy" muscle. An oxygen-deprived muscle is a pain. A muscle gets stiff and sore when its energy supply (glycogen) runs low and lactic acid accumulates. Lactic acid builds up when blood vessels are constricted. Less oxygen goes to the muscle, and waste materials build up which makes the oxygen deprivation even greater. The result can be more acid, less oxygen, and pain. Moderate exercise can help improve the low-oxygen, high-acid ratio.

When muscles are tense or in spasm, one of the biggest advantages of moderate exercise is that your conscious mind figures out pretty quickly that you can move more, and more easily, than you thought you could. Now, there's a positive!

WELLNESS PRINCIPLE: Moderate physical exercise
                      can be a good psychological
                      exercise.

Now let's get down to the nitty-gritty of putting these concepts into practice. It's exercise time.

CHAPTER 8

THE RITE OF EXERCISE

ANYTIME IS EXERCISE TIME

Exercise is just one of the six essentials of health. Unless you are training for competition, the purpose of exercise is to benefit your whole body. It's muscle groups, not just specific muscles such as biceps and abdominals, that long for movement.

Many of us need to make a conscious effort to give our bodies the exercise they deserve. Fortunately, some of the most beneficial exercise is available at home, and it doesn't cost extra. We can walk, stretch, and add a little resistance for muscles to overcome right at home. We don't need expensive equipment to exercise. We have the great outdoors for walking. Inside, we can find elbow room to bend and stretch. Canned foods or books can serve as convenient starter "weights."

Recall the three main health-enhancing benefits of exercise: improved muscle tone and elasticity, enhanced cardiovascular efficiency, and reintegrated neuromuscular communication. Despite all of the complicated exercise programs promoted by books, video tapes, and fitness clinics, walking is the exercise that meets all three criteria with the greatest ease.

Two important reminders.

One: Keep in mind the exercise paradox. We need exercise to be healthy and fit, but exercise can't make you healthy and exercise can't assure health. Health is an inside job. It's a whole-body condition. The objective is for your exercise to be appropri-ate for the level of health of your internal environment. Before you begin any exercise program, check with your health-care professional. This is important for everyone, and it's particularly important if you are a card-carrying couch potato, a high-protein addict, or if you work up a sweat only when the air-conditioner goes off.

Two: Select an exercise that is enjoyable to you. It doesn't make any difference if your cousin enjoys running fifteen miles a week, or your boss is an aerobics nut. The type of exercise you choose is a personal thing. If you don't enjoy what you're doing, you won't do it very long. If you prefer to exercise alone, that's fine. If you prefer a group setting, that's fine too. The big thing is to do something, and do something that's fun. We have enough opportunities in this world to build character by doing things we don't enjoy. You'll get the greatest benefit, both physical and psychological, when pleasure and enthusiasm are active ingredi-ents in your exercise.

WELLNESS PRINCIPLE: Exercise for the fun of it.

WINNING IN A WALK

Walking, done properly, fulfills the three objectives of health-enhancing exercise. The crucial phrase here, is "done properly." A winning walk is one that is purposeful. Erect posture. A well-paced, comfortable stride. No shuffling or mincing about.

WELLNESS PRINCIPLE: Walk with purpose.

Your walk is an advertisement of your attitude as well as your physical condition. Not only does a purposeful stride give your muscles a good no-cost workout but it gives you a greater feeling of confidence. Notice the stride of marching troops, the macho-man, or the runway model. Head up. Firm, extended steps. Fluid, rhythmic motions. By their carriage they exude confidence, energy, and control.

Stand tall when you walk. Give your lungs and other organs room to work. Allow your arms to swing naturally. Remember that your toes bend. You can get from point "A" to point "B" by plopping one foot down then the other without your toes getting into the act. But that limits your stride. Step from heel to toe to propel yourself along. Your stride should be long enough for you to bend those joints between foot and toes.

> WELLNESS PRINCIPLE: Walking is more than put-
>   ting one foot in front of the
>   other.

Purposeful walking offers all three of the benefits of exercise. The muscle-tone and cardiovascular benefits have been well advertised by health professionals and exercise equipment manufacturers. The third benefit of exercise — reintegrating neuromuscular communication — hasn't yet captured the attention of the commercial exercise industry. However, reintegration and re-timing of your internal communication systems is one of the major benefits of walking. That's because well-executed walking is contralateral movement.

Contralateral walking is head-up, relaxed, arm-swinging, comfortable-stride walking. It coordinates movement of opposite sides of the body. This is also called "opposite arm/opposite leg" motion. Left and right sides work in synchronized movement. Right arm swings forward as the left leg extends, and vice versa. That's the way nature intended it.

"Well, certainly," you think. "That's how everyone walks."

But everyone doesn't walk that way. Just about everyone started out walking like that when they were children. But somewhere along the road of life, many people lower their heads, cave in their chests, and "carry" their arms along. Instead of arms swinging naturally at their sides, they are perched stiffly at a quarter-bend. Restricting arm movement isn't "whole-body" walking. It's walking with the feet only. It's a telltale sign of lack of energy, pain, infirmity, or old age — and the person may not be all that old in years.

Walking is a non-competitive, anywhere-sport. Outdoor walking is the most beneficial. Especially when the outdoors is surrounded by nature's beauty and reasonably clean air. Walking in natural surroundings has the added benefit of "feeding the soul." That's a good time to put worry and cares on the back burner and focus on the sights, sounds, and aromas of nature. If you live in a big city where the outside air is saturated with industrial and exhaust pollutants, an enclosed mall may be the cleanest air possible. Mall-walking may not afford the scenic beauty of nature-walking, but it works. And if you are into people-watching or alone-time, a well-populated mall can provide opportunities for either.

Therapeutic, whole-body walking — walking that meets the three purposes of exercise — is most beneficial when you allow your mind to relax. That means tape players and radios with headsets are out. Listening to tapes while walking stimulates the conscious mind. The conscious mind makes judgments about what you are listening to. Those judgments can stimulate subconscious physiological responses that may tense muscles that don't need to be tense. Your exercise period should give your judgmental mind a rest. So instead of listening to tapes while walking, concentrate on the rhythm of your body and the sounds of nature.

How far you walk depends on the shape you're in. That determination is made by your medical doctor or other health care professional. At first, you may become tired after only half-a-block in the city, or a couple of mailboxes in more rural areas. Whatever your endurance level, make sure you leave yourself enough energy to get back to where you started. If you find you are out of breath before you finish your walk, stop and rest. The best length for your walk is however far you can go and still smile and carry on a conversation.

> WELLNESS PRINCIPLE: The activity level of your smile muscles is a good gauge of your energy level.

COMING INTO THE STRETCH

If you are into exercise at all, you know that each exercise session should begin with a warm-up and gentle stretching.

Warming up sends more oxygen-filled blood to muscles. We know that muscles need oxygen to do their jobs. So the first thing muscles need before they can perform at their best is a generous supply of oxygen. An easy warm-up routine increases the blood supply to muscles and primes them for more vigorous activity. A brisk walk or running in place for five minutes or so before exercising gets the heart beating a little faster and sends more oxygen-filled blood to muscles.

> WELLNESS PRINCIPLE: Warm-up to send more blood to muscles.

Warming up allows muscles to stretch more efficiently and reduces the chance of injury.[34] Stretching muscles gently before exercise helps get them ready for strenuous activity. It helps to relax them.

You may think your muscles are relaxed when you start your exercise routine, but they may be more tense than you realize. Muscles respond to the situation of the moment and to the excitement of disturbing thoughts. They contract so you are ready to take action. You can get a good idea of how tense your body is by taking the "shoulder test." It's simple.

The Shoulder Test

Notice, right now, how high your shoulders are. Are they so high that your neck has virtually disappeared? Or are they relaxed and just hanging there where they belong? If your shoulders are up around your ear lobes, your body is tense all over. This is not the ideal state for your body when you exercise. Exercising tension-filled muscles can cause injury. Relax. Consciously relax and let your shoulders drop back to their designed resting position. Taking the shoulder test throughout the day is a good exercise. When you become conscious of the position of your shoulders, you may be surprised to find that they are up much of the time.

WELLNESS PRINCIPLE: When your shoulders are
up-tight, so are you.

OK, so you have your blood flowing, your muscles "warmed up," and your shoulders are in a resting position. Your muscles may be "warmed up," but they may not be quite ready to go. Actually, they are ready to go all the time, but they will go better if they are gently stretched first. Warming-up gets more oxygen to the muscles; stretching affects the working of the muscle. Leaping into strenuous activity without first warming up and stretching can leave you feeling sore the next day, especially if you are just re-activating your exercise life.

In chapter 5, we talked about muscle spindles that are distributed throughout the belly of a muscle. Muscle spindles send information to the nervous system about the length and rate of change of the length of the muscle. When you stretch particular muscles, a status report is sent to central nervous headquarters. That's good. Some coordinating system needs to know what's going on "in the trenches."

But, remember, although the internal body is ever-active and accommodates change, it seeks a steady state — homeostasis, balance. So when a muscle is stretched, its natural tendency is to "recoil" when the stretching is over. The response is rather like that of a stretched elastic band.

Muscles, elastic bands, and we, have a tendency to return to our beginning state after a period of excitement. For example, in our outer macro-life, we are excited by a vacation, or a move, or some other stimulating experience. Then, after the flurry of activity is over we "get back to normal." In our micro-lives, muscles follow much the same pattern. Stretch a muscle and its natural tendency is to contract to "get back to normal." This is called a "stretch reflex." When a muscle is stretched, muscle spindles are "excited." They respond to the excitement of stretching by contracting.

You can notice this reflex when you do "limbering up" exercises, such as bending to touch your toes several times in succession. On the first bend, you can't reach as far as you can on the second. Then, on the third, you can reach a bit farther. There's a reason for this.

In the chapter on muscles, we talked about muscle fibers and their thousands of myosin and actin filaments — the tiny filaments that slide together on cue to contract the muscle. Gentle stretching before energetic stretching primes these tiny filaments to slide apart. Contracted muscle fibers elongate slowly. Muscle fibers are strong, but not indestructible. That's why it's so important that you begin your stretching slowly. No bouncing down to touch your toes. No hard jerks on tense muscles. Jerking or bouncing can injure tiny muscle fibers. And when you injure a lot of muscle fibers, you feel it the next day.

Muscles respond to exercise and they respond to thoughts and emotions. Suppose you spend your life being tense and agitated — ready to do battle or flee. The cues to muscle filaments to contract are constant. This state may be so common for you that you don't even realize consciously that you're tense and that your muscle filaments are nestled snugly together. Nonetheless, off you go for a couple sets of tennis, or a few miles of jogging, or fifty minutes of rhythmical jumping and gyrating with your aerobics class. Mixing strenuous exercise with tense muscles is a sure-fire formula for setting yourself up for stiff, sore muscles.

WELLNESS PRINCIPLE: Jerks irritate tense muscles.

Stretching involves more than muscle spindles and muscle fibers. It involves antagonistic muscles. We can use the familiar example of biceps and triceps of the arm to illustrate this. First, bend one arm at the elbow and feel the muscles of your upper arm with the other hand. Even if you aren't picking up anything, you will feel that your biceps are contracted and triceps relaxed. Now, stretch your arm straight up over your head. Again, with your other hand, feel the muscles of your upper arm. Neither biceps nor triceps are contracted and tight. When you stretch, antagonistic muscles (biceps and triceps) are stretched. Neither is contracted.

The benefits of stretching aren't limited to muscles. Stretching sends updated information on the condition of your muscles to your nervous system.

WELLNESS PRINCIPLE: Stretching is a communica-
                                        tion device.

In order for you to raise your hand (or feel your muscles), you make a conscious decision to do this. You decide to raise your arm with your Red. But your Red doesn't directly signal the actual moving. That's a Green function. And as your arm raises, messages flit back and forth between muscles and Green. Your nervous system is getting updated information on all of this.

You get a side benefit from all of this stretching. Tension relief. When you stretch before or after exercise you don't need to be concerned about the muscles doing their job correctly. You enjoy the feeling of stretching without thinking about what your muscles are doing.

Your nervous system receives muscle information about the stretching. Uniform stretching isn't a defensive posture. Defense requires muscles to be contracted to be ready to do something physical. When antagonistic muscles are stretched, you're not ready to do battle. This state of affairs is not lost on your Green. So stretching can signal your Green that all is right with the world and it can turn off unnecessary defense postures.

> WELLNESS PRINCIPLE: Think about relaxing while
>   you stretch.

The benefits of stretching aren't limited to pre-exercise warm-ups. Stretching after you have finished your routine (whatever it may be) aids the cool-down process.

We know that muscles produce lactic acid when you exercise. Your body gets rid of most of this acid through your lungs. However, when you finish exercising, some of the lactic acid is still in your muscles. After-stretching can help pump some of that acid out of the muscles. And getting rid of the lactic acid helps prevent soreness.[35] So instead of plopping down in a chair after you've exercised strenuously, stretch.

> WELLNESS PRINCIPLE: Stretching gets more than
>   "kinks" out of muscles.

Stretching feels good, can help relax muscles, and can help re-time your internal communication system. However, once again, moderation is the key. Stretching is a gentle movement. You don't increase the benefits of stretching by going at it so hard that you do yourself an injury. If stretching hurts, you're overdoing it. Pain is your body's signal that you've gone too far.

Stretching tight muscles is painful. When you hurt, your body goes defensive. Muscles tighten. That's counterproductive to the benefits of stretching. And the same thing goes for exercising. Exercise doesn't need to be painful to be effective. In fact, you lose many of the benefits of exercise when you tough it out to work through the pain.

> WELLNESS PRINCIPLE: Pain is a warning light on
>   the road to health.

Having said all of that about stretching, it's time to warm up, stretch, and get down to some specifics.

LONG OR STRONG

As was pointed out at the beginning of this book, this isn't your usual exercise manual. The focus here is on whole-body health. It's not a build-bigger-muscles-and-flatten-your-stomach book. Exercise is only one essential of a healthy lifestyle. The goal is to help you make choices about exercise that will be of the greatest benefit to you personally. There's no one absolutely perfect exercise for everyone. Even walking — the most universally beneficial exercise of all — isn't possible for everyone. Yet just about everyone who can move can exercise somehow. The objective is to help you reach your own personal highest potential level of health. Young, old, and those in the awkward in-between years can reap whole health benefits — physical, physiological, emotional, and mental — from exercise.

> WELLNESS PRINCIPLE: Age is not a ticket to
> inactivity.

Exercise is a life-long activity. Certainly, age is a factor in more aggressive sports such as football and bull riding. But bone-busting potential doesn't add to the whole-body benefits of exercise. And since we're talking whole-body health, not about training for an upcoming pentathlon, the suggestions for exercises here are suitable for all ages. However, once again, be sure to check with your doctor before you increase your exercise level.

Exercising as a part of whole-body health means different things for various ages. We may not be able to sustain the speed, endurance and agility of children as we age. But that doesn't mean that we are destined for increasing frailty. The more correct choices we make in the six essentials, the longer we can look forward to active, vibrant, fulfilling lives. We continue to make essential choices throughout life. We don't have six essentials until we reach a particular age, then drop the exercise essential. Exercise is as important in later years as it is in youth.

"Later years" is a purposely vague time of life. Some of us reach "later years" in our forties. Others don't get there until several decades later. So gauge the choices in your exercise essential to fit your stage of life and your interests. Start slowly and keep at it. Before long you will find that endurance and strength pick up.

WELLNESS PRINCIPLE: Exercise according to your stage in life, not your age in life.

Recall that we talked about how cells can turn glucose into energy either aerobically (with the help of oxygen) or anaerobically (without the help of oxygen). Aerobic processes supply energy for long term exercises; anaerobic processes are for short bursts of energy. Aerobic and anaerobic processes can be related to the two major types of exercise: endurance exercises, and resistance, or weight-training, exercises.

Endurance exercises, such as jogging, are the heavy-sweat producing activities that increase your heart rate and send more oxygen-filled blood coursing through your veins. To get this additional oxygen to muscles the heart and lungs work faster and harder. The heart muscle, and the circulatory system in general, are strengthened. The lungs (or pulmonary system) get a more intense workout than usual. And, of course, all of this is in response to a direct need of the muscles which are also working hard. Endurance exercises are great whole-body exercises. However, endurance exercises may not dramatically increase muscle strength. Take swimming, for instance. Swimming can increase muscle strength slightly. However, top level swimmers use resistance exercises outside the water to strengthen their muscles.

Resistance exercises, such as weight lifting and push-ups, are the grunt-and-groan activities that increase muscle strength.

Most sports are combinations of the two. Tennis, for example, is a lot of running (aerobic) punctuated with bursts of ball-returning muscle power (anaerobic). Basketball is a lot of running (aerobic) punctuated with leaps and quick ball deliveries (anaerobic). Even golf that uses anaerobic processes for the two-second swing can include aerobic benefits if the player walks the course rather than riding a cart.

Swimming sprints may leave the swimmer huffing and puffing. But short sprints lean toward the burst-of-speed anaerobic side. Distance or lap swimming brings in aerobic benefits (without the sweat).

Both endurance and resistance exercises can strengthen muscles and increase flexibility. But it takes time and repetition.

WELLNESS PRINCIPLE: In general, endurance exercises are aerobic, and resistance exercises are anaerobic.

So, which is the best type of exercise for you?

In the long run, the most beneficial exercise is a combination of endurance and resistance. However, don't pull on the athletic shoes and make a nose-holding jump into a sea of frantic workouts yet. The first step is to devise an exercise program that you consider fun. If it isn't fun, it's a chore and will be short-lived. The second step is to check with your doctor to see that your version of exercise fun is compatible with your particular state of health. Consider where you are in the health, stamina, and strength departments. It took time for you to develop, or undermine, your current health, stamina, and strength. If any of them is underdeveloped, it will take time for them to gradually increase.

WELLNESS PRINCIPLE: Health-enhancing exercise
isn't a quick fix.

EXERCISE THROUGH THE AGES

We came with a complete set of muscles at birth. Before and
after we were born, we moved and we stretched, and we pushed
against whatever was available. We worked our muscles, and
they grew bigger and stronger. It wasn't a conscious act. We
didn't consciously work at strengthening muscles so we could
control our heads, legs, feet, arms, and hands. We just kept
moving. And with movement and resistance to movement,
muscles grew bigger and stronger.

WELLNESS PRINCIPLE: Building muscle doesn't
take thought; it takes action.

Generally, muscles get larger until early adulthood. Then, if
physical activity slacks off and the lifestyle is relatively sedentary, muscle fibers begin to shrink. Fat takes their place. And, if
this continues, by the time we're about 80 years old, we've lost
20 to 40 percent of our muscle mass.[36]

We may not be able to completely stem the loss of muscle
mass as the years go by. However, we can keep moving and
stretching and pushing against things to slow the process and
retain as much vitality as possible. Studies have shown that
weight-training programs can help 80- and 90-year-olds to build
muscle mass and improve mobility. And, as a positive side effect,
mental agility improves along with physical agility.[37] Not a bad
deal at all. But the positive doesn't end there. There's the bone
factor.

Bones are made up primarily of organic and inorganic
materials. The organic is chiefly a protein called collagen. This
is laid down in the form of fibers and give bones toughness. The
inorganic material is principally calcium salts that give bones
hardness and rigidity. And, surprise, bones also contain a small

amount of water.[38] So the old "dry bones" bit isn't completely accurate.

> WELLNESS PRINCIPLE: Your bones are alive; help
>   keep them well.

We tend to think of the bones that make up our skeletal system as our rock solid support system. However, the bones you have today are not exactly the same bones you had yesterday. Bone is continually lost and replaced. Bone cells are absorbed and new cells deposited.[39]

The comings and goings of bone cells are nearly equal, so the overall bone mass stays relatively constant.[40] However, bones adapt to need. They respond to the stress put on them. Bones thicken when they must habitually support heavy loads. And they adapt their shape and strength to accommodate to stress patterns.[41] That's why the bones of athletes are generally heavier than the bones of career TV channel surfers. Bone growth is determined by structural needs.[42] Lifting and pushing are stresses to bones. Walking, running, lifting, and other activities that put moderate stress on bones help them to get stronger.

> WELLNESS PRINCIPLE: Help strengthen your bones
>   — dig a garden, rake leaves,
>   clean out the garage.

As the years go by, continuing to bend, stretch, and push against things can help strengthen bones. Bone-strengthening isn't limited to the young. As we age, we need to keep our bones in the best shape possible. The old brittle bone problem that seems to be synonymous with aging in our country isn't necessarily inevitable. Indeed, the trend for bone loss and brittleness increases with age. That's because the mineral content of bones (the hard part) increases, and the organic content (the elasticity and toughness part) decreases. However, studies have shown that women as old as 70 can slightly increase their bone density by lifting weights.[43] This isn't an overnight improvement, but if you're going to live to a vigorous old age, you may as well keep your bones as strong as possible.

For muscles and bones that have been on vacation for years, resistance, or weight-training, can help strengthen them. The resistance doesn't need to be tremendous. Weights as light as a pound give the muscles something to work against. As strength increases, the weights can be a little heavier. The objective is to put moderate stress on both muscles and bones. As strength and endurance gradually build, the amount of stress can be gradually increased.

> WELLNESS PRINCIPLE: You're never too old (or too young) to start exercising.

EXERCISE THAT FITS
Your exercise program should fit your personal circumstances and needs. Whether you are beginning to exercise or have been at it for years, the objectives for health are the same. Bones and muscles come with basic structures and dynamics for everyone. The difference between exercise for the beginner and veteran is in intensity and endurance.

With that in mind, let's have a quick review of the better-health objectives and benefits of exercising regularly. Remember, we're into whole-body health, not body-building.

Regular, moderate exercise can:
>   Enhance cardiorespiratory efficiency — physical and
>   physiological benefit
>   Improve muscle tone and elasticity — physical and
>   physiological benefit
>   Reintegrate neuromuscular (mind-body) communication
>   — physical, physiological, mental, and emotional
>   benefits

Exercises that include all three of these benefits are ideal, whole-body exercises. Contralateral walking, jogging, running, aerobic dancing, and other exercises that get the heart pumping faster, the muscles moving, and integrate movement of opposite sides of the body come closest to the ideal category. You don't need expensive equipment for any of these exercise programs. However, your own personal circumstances should be considered in selecting the exercise best for you.

Some exercises require blocks of time to be effective. Others can be interspersed with your activities throughout the day. For many people, finding a place to walk may be a problem. Jogging and running are high-impact joint-jolters — ankles, knees, and hips take quite a pounding that may lead to injury and pain. Aerobic dancing can be done in a group setting or at home. The group usually meets someplace that requires traveling to get there. At-home aerobics that are generally solitary sessions done with a video as a leader, often become a drudge.

WELLNESS PRINCIPLE: Drudgery is not motivation
                                          for long-term commitment.

The exercises that provide the greatest whole-health benefits are those that coordinate both sides, upper and lower portions, and move as many muscles and joints as possible through their full range of motion. And now, instead of just talking about exercise, let's get on with it.

CHAPTER 9

ROAM YOUR RANGE OF MOTION

DESIGNED TO MOVE

Each of us is an assembly of hinges and springs energized by physiological power plants. Our muscles and other systems respond to signals that originate in the Red, Yellow, or Green. We are designed to move.

Our moveable parts have minimum and maximum capacities. We adjust the rate and intensity of movement to fit the needs of the moment. And our physiological mechanisms work better and become stronger when their parts are periodically allowed to work to their greatest capacity. Internal systems, organs, and muscles can work at variable speeds. But they need to be allowed to reach their maximum capacity regularly. It's the old "use it or lose it" syndrome.

> WELLNESS PRINCIPLE: Your body was designed for
> maximum performance.

Aerobic exercises push your heart and lungs to work harder than they do when you're taking a stroll in the park. Sports and other exercises call on muscles and connective tissue to stretch out and power up. When you push your body beyond its normal work-day physical activity level, you move muscles beyond their

habit zone. Of course, if you're a professional athlete, construction worker, walking postal carrier, farmer, or regular in another
physically demanding job, muscles get a pretty good workout
nearly every day. However, if you lead that kind of life, you
probably don't sit around reading books on the health benefits
and glories of exercise.

The great majority of Americans are considerably less
physically active than the aforementioned subgroups. For
millions of Americans, muscle and joint activity settles into a
comfortable, but limited, pattern of movement. It's not that
muscles and joints can't move more, it's that they are rarely
called on to extend themselves. As a result, in time, their range
of motion can become limited. One of the objectives of exercise
is to allow muscles and joints to once again reach their full range
of motion.

The term "range of motion" is generally applied to the amount
of movement possible for a joint or joints. Yet your bones can't
move by themselves. For controlled movement, either you or
someone else must provide energy and direction. In either case,
it's your bones, muscles, tendons, and ligaments that are involved in your movement. For example, if you break an arm or
leg, usually the broken bone is immobilized. Its range of motion
is limited. During the healing process, a physical therapist may
help to move the injured limb to the outer limits of its diminished
range of motion. The objective is to keep expanding movement
until the pre-injury full range of motion is again possible.

But it doesn't take a broken bone or other injury to reduce the
range of motion of joints and muscles. Inactivity can have the
same effect. That's often demonstrated after sitting in one
position for a while. You get up and, for first step or two, fluidity
of movement is missing. Or stay in bed for a couple of days, and
you become "weak." And, as we saw in the story of the patient
with tense but flabby muscles, range of motion can also be
limited by emotional stress. A combination of inactivity and
stress can be a powerful motion inhibitor.

WELLNESS PRINCIPLE: Up-tight recliner-jockeys
                                        limit their range of motion.

We have seen how emotions can affect the body. Emotions
such as anger, fear, or guilt keep your body in defense — up-
tight. Muscles are contracted and ready to explode into action
which may or may not happen. Muscle contraction is only one
part of movement. For fluid movement, as one muscle contracts,
its opposite number must relax. They work cooperatively. We
used the example of the biceps and triceps. To lift your coffee
cup to your mouth, your biceps (at the front of your upper arm)
contract while your triceps (at the back of your upper arm) relax.
But if the triceps don't relax, the muscles work against each
other.

And we may not always realize that some muscles aren't
cooperating with their counterparts. The Arm-Swing Test can be
a good indicator.

Arm-Swing Test
Stand in front of a mirror. Raise your right arm straight out to
shoulder height — or as close to shoulder height as you can get
it. Relax your wrist so that your hand flops down naturally at the
end of your outstretched arm. Now, keep your elbow straight and
let your arm swing from your shoulder. Don't guide it, slow it
down, or direct it. Let gravity take over and the weight of your
hand will pull down your arm.

Notice in the mirror what happened when your arm
swings down to your side. Does it swing backward past
your hips then come back toward the front like a sideways
pendulum? Or does it get to your side and stop abruptly?

If your muscles are loose and relaxed in response to
your conscious Red intent, your arm should swing loosely
past your hip.

If your arm didn't make it past your hip, your muscles
are working against themselves without you realizing it.

They are maintaining tension they don't need at the moment. They aren't doing anything wrong. They're performing correct functions at an inappropriate time. It's a timing problem — Yellow override.

We talked earlier about timing. As a refresher, timing is more than keeping the beat of toe-tapping music or a rhythmic swimming stroke. Timing refers to your body performing correct functions at appropriate times. A timing problem is the body performing correct functions at inappropriate times. Common timing problems can show up as the digestive system running full-tilt when there's no food around to digest, or blood pressure rising to a non-occasion. Similarly, if muscles are overly tense and contracted when they should be relaxed, that's a timing problem.

> WELLNESS PRINCIPLE: Your body can't do
> anything wrong, but it can
> do a right thing at an inap-
> propriate time.

Here's another quick exercise that can indicate that muscles are tense and contracted at an inappropriate time. This one involves your legs rather than your arms. Your success at this "test" also indicates your general flexibility.

The Squat Test

Stand with your weight evenly balanced and your feet about six inches apart. Now, without holding on to anything, squat down on your heels. The first question is: Can you get all the way down so that your buttocks are on your heels? The second question is: Can you get all the way down and keep your heels on the floor, or do your heels come up so that you are balancing on your toes?

If you can squat down and keep your heels on the floor without falling over backwards, the opposing muscles in your legs are relaxing evenly. If you can't squat, or if your heels come up off the floor, or if you fall backwards, muscles that should be relaxed aren't. Muscle tone and timing are inappropriate.

The squat test is an *indicator* of muscle tone. If you can get all the way down to a squat and keep your heels on the floor, the indication is that the muscles needed to perform this maneuver are neither too tense nor too loose. If you can squat all the way down but your heels come off the floor, the indication is that excess tension in some muscles is keeping them from relaxing fully. Not being able to squat much at all is an indicator that most of your muscles are overly tense. If muscles are more than slightly tense, movement is inhibited. Muscles that need to relax so you can make the complete descent don't let go.

Keep in mind that muscles are supposed to be able to contract and relax. They don't need to be contracted all the time. So a "failed" squat test is an indicator that something is keeping some muscles tense when they don't need to be. The muscles are functioning correctly (contracting) at an inappropriate time. It's a timing problem. And timing problems begin with interference.

INTERFERING WITH THE DESIGN

We are designed to move. We do so with amazing agility and ease in our youth. However, for the most part, even the "physically fit" find that their movements become less fluid and dynamic as the years go by. The Arm Swing Test and Squat Test are indicators of restricted movement. And restricted movement in a "healthy body" can be seen as toning and timing problems.

We talked about muscle tone in Chapter muscles.sr2. Muscle tone is the steady state of slight contraction. Muscle tone helps your body resist the pull of gravity. It's the muscles' ability to resist a force without changing length. Among other benefits, muscle tone keeps your back straight when you're standing up, and your mouth closed when it's not being used. The best muscle tone is just the amount of tension needed to do the particular job at hand. Not too much and not too little. If muscles stay tensed more than necessary to do their job, they become tired. If they are too relaxed, they can't do their job effectively. They are flabby.

WELLNESS PRINCIPLE: Muscle tone is consistent slight tension.

Muscle tone affects how you do the squat test. Muscle tone is a Green function. Your subconscious Green keeps just the right amount of subtle tension on particular muscles as needed.

Muscles respond to Green instructions. Green bases these instructions on information received from two sources: signals from conscious Red, and signals from non-conscious Yellow. Green instructions are always correct and perfect. However, Red and Yellow information may not be. So inappropriate muscle tone starts in Red or Yellow.

In the squat test situation, the decision to squat was made in the Red. So if muscles are more tense than they need to be and you can't squat down completely, it's not Red that's interfering with the process — it's Yellow.

Your Yellow is your experience storehouse crammed full of learned responses.

Your Yellow is very powerful and it's always with you. It helps you respond to commonplace stimuli without relearning each response. For example, it's your Yellow that drives your car for you. You don't consciously think about exactly how far to turn the wheel to avoid that pothole in the road. You learned that when you first started driving. The amount of turn you need to make is a learned response stored in your Yellow.

Your Yellow has also learned that day-to-day situations can be filled with "danger." And if your Yellow is "filled" with "danger" signals, your Green gets the message. Green responds to messages; it doesn't evaluate the necessity for the messages. It makes no difference to your Green if the message is accurate or inaccurate. The Green response is perfect. So if your muscles are overly tense when they don't need to be, it's your Yellow that's overlaying "danger" signals appropriate to past situations onto current events that are not dangerous. Yellow is sending "danger" signals to your Green, so Green responds by keeping muscles prepared to run or fight. Yellow override. Your muscles are responding correctly to Green signals prompted by Yellow memories instead of actual current conditions. And memories originate with thoughts and emotions attached to past experiences.

> WELLNESS PRINCIPLE: Memories of the past can interfere with present muscle tone.

Does that mean that you are doomed to ill-timed tense muscles and inappropriate responses for the rest of your life? Not at all.

It means that you can now recognize that some physical limitations may not be physical in origin. It also means that if inappropriate timing is keeping you from being as limber and comfortable as you would like, you may be able to do something about it. If past thoughts can keep you up-tight, you can re-program your Yellow to respond to more appropriate current conditions. You can't "erase" memories, but memory is constantly being "reconstructed" through fresh input. You can adjust the stimuli to which your body responds to be more in keeping with current conditions. That's good news.

STEP ALONG FOR RETIMING
Inappropriate timing that affects muscles and keeps them contracted, tense, and ready to go, prevents them from relaxing. And since timing is a function of past and present thoughts and attitudes, you can do something about it. You don't have control over the past, but you have control over your current thoughts

and attitudes, including current attitudes toward past experiences.

In my opinion, one of the biggest "scientific breakthroughs" of the twenty-first century will be acceptance by the "scientific community" of the concept that thoughts and attitudes are the greatest threat to health. Physiology disturbing thoughts, attitudes, and emotions can cause more havoc in the human body than germs, genetics, fat, and inactivity combined.

Conscious thoughts conjured up by your Red generally focus on present trauma and turmoil — family problems, financial shortfalls, personal affronts and inadequacies, political, moral, and ethical biases, and the like. Your physiology responds to these.

But memories can also influence physiology. Memories, along with their attached physiology-affecting emotions, stored in your Yellow are ever-present and easily triggered. It doesn't take much to keep Yellow inspired physiological responses going. Current thoughts and emotions that contain a hint of a similar past incident can perpetuate Yellow override. And since our thinking tends to follow habitual patterns, we constantly relate the now to the past. That's why it is so important for you to saturate your mind with relaxing, positive thoughts when you are walking. Focused, therapeutic walking — or exercise of any kind — is more whole-body beneficial when your thoughts aren't interfering with your physiology.

WELLNESS PRINCIPLE: Positive thoughts help to
neutralize the negative
stored in your Yellow.

Your thoughts are one of the biggest — if not the ultimate biggest — influence on your physiology. We might say that "thoughts" are the energy stimulus and "physiology" is the active response. So combining thoughts with action can help to retime responses to inappropriate Yellow memories. Focused walking is an excellent combination of thoughts and action. Mentally focus on pleasant positive thoughts while you walk.

The best place to do this is in pleasant natural surroundings where the air is fresh and the sights and sounds of nature stimulate your senses.

Realistically, many people are hard pressed to find "pleasant natural surroundings" that are ideal for a good retiming walk. While pleasant natural surroundings can enhance your retiming walk, the setting isn't as important as the process. Mall-walking may be the most secure setting for many people. Any place you are safe and comfortable is fine. Retiming benefits are determined by how you walk and how you think while you are walking, not by where you walk.

In chapter 8, we talked about the head-up, arm-swinging, right leg-left arm, left leg-right arm purposeful stride walking of contralateral movements. Contralateral walking is whole-body walking. This action gets the heart beating a little faster, the breathing a little deeper, and the neuromuscular system in synch. The greatest benefit of contralateral walking comes when you allow your body to be as balanced as possible. Carrying something in your hands or slung over your shoulder throws off the natural balance of the body. Walking your dog may or may not allow balanced contralateral walking. In a rural setting, perhaps your dog can walk freely with you. In an urban setting, where your dog is on a leash, the contralateral effect can be disturbed. The occasional pulling and tugging on the leash by an energetic pet can interfere with your rhythmical balance.

WELLNESS PRINCIPLE: Contralateral walking is a
balancing act.

Once you have determined that you are going to walk and where you are going to do it, the next questions are how much, how fast, and how far.

Exercise/fitness gurus have conditioned us to accept that we need thirty or more sweat producing minutes of exercise five days a week to achieve good looks, glistening hair, charming personality, and high-level success. Well, maybe those aren't the exact claims. But the general consensus has been that to be effective for either weight-loss or shaping-up, exercise regimens should include regular and frequent periods of concentrated exertion.

More recent findings indicate that breaking down long, intense periods into shorter periods of varying intensity can be beneficial.[44] Translated into walking, you don't need to put in forty-five minutes of high intensity walking five days a week to reap health-enhancing benefits. Sessions of about thirty minutes that include periods of easy walking and fast walking give you a variety of benefits.

Walking is multi-beneficial when you start out at a comfortable pace for about ten minutes, put on the steam for the next ten minutes, then cruise home at comfort level for the last ten minutes.

When you walk at a comfortable pace for about ten minutes, your body uses anaerobic (without oxygen) and aerobic (with oxygen) processes. We talked earlier about how the body uses energy from anaerobic activity for power moves and to get us off to a fast start. This instant energy comes from carbohydrates stored in cells and leaves lactic acid as a by-product. Sustained activity calls on aerobic processes that use oxygen to convert carbohydrates, and ultimately fats, as "fuel" to produce energy.

When you speed up your walk, your heart rate and breathing intensify as energy production switches to aerobic processes. This gets your blood scurrying through your veins to soak up as much oxygen as possible and to get rid of physiological acid. You can go a lot faster and farther on aerobically produced energy than you can on anaerobic energy. Aerobic fast walking exercises both your cardiovascular system and your muscles. It helps build endurance. When you slow down again, your body has a chance to "work out" the lactic acid that muscles have been producing and you lessen the chance of next-day soreness. Begin and end your outing with ten minutes of warm-up and cool-down walking.

WELLNESS PRINCIPLE: Fast walking benefits your cardiovascular system.

While fast walking helps strengthen your blood and oxygen delivery systems, easy contralateral walking helps retime internal communications. In contralateral walking, all sections of the body are coordinated to work in balanced unity — left and right, top and bottom. Opposing muscles contract and relax in synchronized rhythm. Neither sympathetic nor parasympathetic nervous system is over stressed. Internal "message circuits" are freed of "clutter." All of this means that sessions that include both fast and slow walking improve muscle tone and elasticity and internal timing.

And there's more.

We generally think of hard, sweat-generating, heart-pounding, strained-expression type exercises as the master fat burners. And, indeed, they are. However, one researcher found that leisurely walking can reap fat burning benefits. He divided the participants into three groups. Each group walked three miles a day for twenty-four days. One group walked at an easy pace of 20 minutes per mile. The second group kept a brisk pace of 15 minutes per mile. And the third group stepped out at a serious walking rate of 12 minutes per mile. As expected, the faster groups improved more in endurance and overall fitness. However, surprisingly, the slowest group used the highest proportion of calories from fat.[45] So, easy walking burns fat. How's that for a day-brightener! But a word of caution: fat-burning easy-walking takes more than leisurely strolls to the refrigerator or snack cupboard during TV commercials to be effective. You need to "go the distance" — miles rather than feet.

WELLNESS PRINCIPLE: Easy walking can be a fat

burner.

How far or long you can exercise safely depends on your overall physical condition. One thing is certain, however: If you have been a card-carrying lounge chair jockey your muscle tone and endurance level aren't very high. So before you sign up for the "Advanced Aerobics for Beautiful People" class at your local fitness center and run out to buy the latest in fashionable exercise togs, check with your doctor, and begin to get yourself in shape with some elementary stretching and walking.

The first rule for walking is: Stretch before you walk, and walk only until you begin to get tired.

Stretching helps to loosen and warm-up muscles. Your chances of muscle injury are reduced when you ease them into uncharacteristic activity. It doesn't take much exertion of semi-dormant muscles to make them sore the next day. Stretching before and after exercise can go a long way to avoid the morning after "Oh, I'm so stiff" syndrome.

And if you are walking around your neighborhood, be sure that you don't go so far afield that you must struggle to get back. Pace yourself.

WELLNESS PRINCIPLE: A mixture of fast and slow
                      gives all systems a chance
                      to go.

One of the unsung benefits of therapeutic contralateral walking is that it is economical. No expensive equipment needed. All you need is a pair of good, comfortable shoes with well-cushioned soles. And the only reason you need those is because you are probably walking in our modern jungle instead of nature's jungle that is considerably softer. People walked quite well without shoes for thousands of years. The skin on the soles of their feet became quite tough. But since the soles of the feet of most of us are rarely in direct contact with anything more rugged than a carpet, most of us fall into the tenderfoot category and need shoes.

The two requirements for therapeutic walking are (1) an O.K. from your doctor, and (2) good shoes.

Again, a reminder to check with your doctor before you launch any exercise program — even a program as natural as walking.

Contralateral walking on a thirty-minute outing is good overall exercise, but it probably doesn't give muscles and joints a full workout. Muscles and joints don't extend through their full range of motion. And, of course, I wouldn't bring this up without telling you why full range of motion is important, and offering an alternative. In the next chapter, we'll look at an exercise you can do at home that not only takes your muscles and joints through their full range of motion and fulfills the three objectives, but feels good in the process. However, we'll take a look at *why* full-range-of-motion exercise is an important ingredient in any exercise program.

FULL RANGE OF MOTION

Full range of motion usually refers to freedom of joint movement. However, since muscles and other soft tissue are involved in moving a joint, we will use the term "full range of motion" to refer to both joint and muscle action.

Full range of motion exercises are important because they give muscles a chance to fully contract and fully relax. Muscles stretch more easily when they are relaxed. Stretch a contracted muscle and later you may feel stiff and sore. Stretching a *relaxed* muscle through its full range of motion is as important as contracting it to its maximum. The object of full range of motion movement is to coordinate and retime groups of muscles, not to strengthen a particular muscle.

WELLNESS PRINCIPLE: Enjoy the freedom of a full
range of motion.

When you stretch a muscle it wants to return to its original position. Actually, muscles don't "want" to do anything. Muscles don't think. They don't decide to shrink or grow or hurt or just sit there. All they can do is respond to signals from your Green to contract or relax. Nonetheless, when a muscle is stretched, its response is to contract back to its original tension. A short refresher on how muscles know when to relax or contract might be helpful.

The Green subconscious knows what muscles are doing all the time. Some of this information comes from muscle spindles which are tiny structures within the muscles themselves. Muscle spindles detect and signal relative muscle length. Other information comes from Golgi tendon organs which are tiny organs of the tendons. Golgi tendon organs detect and signal muscle tension.

When a muscle is stretched, or elongated, muscle spindles in the belly of the muscle send information through the spinal cord to the cerebellum about the muscle length or rate of change in muscle length. The more the spindle is stretched, the faster it sends signals to the subconscious. This information is used by the subconscious to adjust muscle movements. Rapid-fire transmission of information allows smooth movements when you walk, throw a baseball, or perform other coordinated feats. The information is also used to keep muscle activity within a safe range to prevent injuries. Violent stretching or overstretching can injure the muscle. And the body has a built-in bias against being injured. Injuries reduce chances of survival. So we have protection responses known as "stretch reflexes." Stretch reflexes cause reflex contraction of stretched muscles.

Stretch reflexes come in four types: dynamic, static, negative, and load.

The dynamic stretch reflex causes an instantaneous, strong contraction of a muscle that is stretched suddenly. The dynamic stretch reflex is immediate, short, and strong.

The static stretch reflex lasts longer. It opposes the force that is causing the excess length of the muscle. The static reflex keeps the muscle slightly contracted as long as it is elongated.

The negative stretch reflex works in the opposite way. It opposes the shortening of the muscle the way the positive stretch reflex opposes the lengthening of the muscle.

The load reflex limits the downward movement of the forearm when a heavy weight, such as a bowling ball, is put into the hand.

Stretch reflexes help muscles maintain the status quo.[46] And it all happens without conscious thought.

> WELLNESS PRINCIPLE: Stretching is a body-mind exercise.

Stretching involves the full muscle as well as the small belly of the muscle. So stretching involves the complete muscle as well as communication with the cerebellum. Since one of the major purposes of exercise is to reintegrate neuromuscular communication — that is, improve mind-body "dialogue" — you benefit from exercises that include controlled stretching. Yoga and tai chi exercises are good examples of controlled stretching.

In tai chi exercises, large muscle groups are used to perform slow, smooth, graceful movements. The whole body is involved. Controlled breathing, mental attitudes, and eye movements are incorporated with physical motion. Not only is the whole body involved, the whole body benefits.[47]

Since yoga, tai chi, and other Eastern-culture exercises have stood the test of time for generations, they must have something going for them. They are dynamic without being violent, slam-bang, muscle abusers. And they include full range of motion plus mental discipline.

> WELLNESS PRINCIPLE: Health is not achieved by physical activity alone.

So, am I suggesting that you charge off to your nearest yoga or tai chi instruction centers?

Well, you can if that's what turns your crank. And it would probably do wonders for your physical and mental well-being. However, you can reap many of the same benefits by a western version of controlled movement, stretching, relaxing, and breathing that you can learn and do right at home — the Morter March.

CHAPTER 10

MARCH TOWARD HEALTH

STRETCH TO RETIME

The Morter March might be seen as a miniature version of strenuous aerobic exercise. For most people, only a few repetitions are needed to increase heart rate, deepen breathing, and begin to tire muscles. Yet, the movements are deliberate and smooth which gives the added benefit of improved balance. The Morter March helps to improve neurological balance — re-time internal communication — by extending large muscle groups and their joints through a full range of motion. You can do this exercise as a part of your regular slow-fast-slow walk outside, and you can do it independently. However, as you will see, the movements of this exercise might appear a bit strange to the casual observer. So, if you are overly concerned with what the neighbors think, you may be more comfortable doing it within the privacy of your own home before you go out where the neighbors can see you.

In the Morter March, you move muscles just beyond their comfort zone. No one else knows how far you can bend or stretch without causing pain or doing yourself an injury. You are the only one. Your present comfort zone is your "habit zone." Your habit zone is the range of motion your muscles and joints find most comfortable. We all have fairly well defined daily routines that require particular physical movements. Over time, muscles can settle into a comfortable but limited routine of movements. This exercise, like yoga and tai chi, gives you and your muscles an opportunity to move beyond the customary habit zone. You stretch, relax, and re-time at the same time.

WELLNESS PRINCIPLE: Allow your muscles to express their full potential — broaden your habit zone.

The Morter March
Stand comfortably erect. Alert yet relaxed.

Take an extended step with your left foot, keeping your back (right) foot firmly on the floor. Stretch just far enough forward with your left foot so that you can keep the heel of your back (right) foot on the floor.

As you extend your left leg, raise your right arm to about a 45 degree angle. Your left arm will automatically move back to help you balance. Stretch your left arm downward behind you at about a 45 degree angle. Your position at this point is left leg and right arm stretched forward, right leg and left arm stretched back.

Now, turn your head toward the side of the extended right arm, look up, and s-t-r-e-t-c-h.

While you are in your extended position, take a deep breath and hold both your breath and position for five to ten seconds.

Exhale and repeat the maneuver with the opposite leg and arm.

Repeat the sequence three or four times — fewer, if you become tired.

Do the Morter March "workout" twice a day.

You can also do this exercise as a continuous motion — without the breath-holding — at the beginning and end of your 30-minute walk. Two Morter March steps with each foot are enough. You will notice that the movements are exaggerations of a normal contralateral walk.

When you first attempt the Morter March, you may find that you have trouble balancing in your extended position. You can improve your stability by giving yourself as broad a base on which to stand as you need. Rather than putting one foot on a line directly in front of the other, widen your stance (sideways) to suit your balance needs. You will probably find after your have done this exercise regularly for a week or so that your balance has improved. Then you can narrow your stance to fit your improved balancing skills.

Make sure you do the Morter March with contralateral movement — extend right leg and left arm simultaneously and left leg and right arm simultaneously. Some patients find that their initial inclination is to step out on one leg and have the arm on the same side follow. That's backwards. If you extend the same-side arm and leg simultaneously (i.e., right leg/right arm), you may find you develop a headache, neck ache, or other ache.

When correctly done, the Morter March is a very powerful retiming exercise. Patients have reported that after doing the Morter March they find they have more flexibility, feel more energetic, and seem to be more "put together." The length of time required for changes to be noticeable depends on the individual. Some people are "reasonably healthy" when they begin. They may notice changes quickly. Others are "unreasonably un-healthy." They may not notice any difference for weeks or months.

FULL RANGE OF BENEFITS
Your current physical condition will determine how well you are able to do the Morter March and how far you can step and stretch. Some people will be able to move more easily, step further, reach further, and hold their position and breath more easily than others. How long you can hold your stretched position will depend on your balance. We each have our own present

degree of balance, agility, flexibility, and endurance. The degree doesn't matter. The Morter March uses such a wide range of systems that over a period of time balance, agility, flexibility, and endurance can improve.

Stretching is the key. Start out easily. Stretch just enough so that you can begin to feel tension in the muscles; then quit. Although you may not be able to stretch as much as you think you should able to, as long as you reach your personal maximum, stretching has beneficial effects. When muscles are stretched, their activity increases. Muscle metabolism is stepped up. When metabolism speeds up, more energy and more acid are produced.

It may take a few days for acid that has accumulated in muscles to dissipate. As acid is "squeezed out" of muscles, they won't be as painful, and your endurance will be greater. With diligence, these improvements come quickly. You will probably notice a difference in about ten days.

WELLNESS PRINCIPLE: Stretching increases muscle
metabolism.

In addition to improving balance, agility, and endurance, stretching also opens the way for neuromuscular communication to be retimed. We might compare stretching muscles to taking the kinks out of a garden hose. When a kinked hose is stretched out straight, the passageway is opened and as much water as the hose can carry flows freely.

We can carry the hose analogy a step further. Even though the kinks are gone and the water flows freely, the hose isn't flimsy and floppy. It's firm but flexible. And it carries the maximum amount of water energy along at maximum speed. When muscles are stretched to the outer limit of their comfort range, internal communication energy can flow more freely.

Stretching involves the whole length of the muscle as well as the muscle spindles in the muscle's belly. So stretching communicates with the cerebellum. In the process, your Green becomes more aware of a muscle that may have a residual resting tone higher than normal. That's where the retiming comes in.

If the muscles are contracted at an inappropriate time in response to Yellow override, then the residual resting tone of muscles is stronger than is appropriate for current conditions. The muscles are doing a correct thing at an inappropriate time. Stretching sends updated messages to the Green (cerebellum). And since your Green doesn't analyze or judge, it responds to the update.

WELLNESS PRINCIPLE: Muscles are retimed during
                                        the stretching phase.

An important retiming ingredient in the Morter March is "take a deep breath and hold it."

We know that cells require a constant supply of oxygen and that muscles use a lot of oxygen when they work. Consequently, when you stretch some muscles and tense others, a lot of oxygen is required. But if you are holding your breath, the oxygen supply is limited. So what happens?

As far as your Green is concerned, a survival crisis situation is escalating. The oxygen supply doesn't meet the need. But your Green is resourceful. It will "de-activate" any physiological processes not needed for immediate survival, and muscles use a lot of oxygen just to stay tense. So, muscles that aren't actively involved in keeping you upright at the moment, relax. With muscles relaxed, a few more seconds of life-sustaining oxygen are available. It's a survival mechanism.

However, muscles aren't the greatest oxygen consumers. The brain holds that distinction. And the brain is active all the time. Yet if your body needs oxygen to survive, even unnecessary brain activity can be curtailed. Brain activity that is using a lot of oxygen in response to current emotions such as worry, is put on "hold." Worry, anger, and frustration are counterproductive to immediate survival.

WELLNESS PRINCIPLE: Negative emotions are
oxygen-eaters.

The Morter March also gives muscle groups the benefit of
being contracted. Muscles are retoned during the contractive
phase. Muscles are designed to contract. That's their job. They
contract to overcome resistance. Moving weight around, be it
your own body mass, the refrigerator, or a five pound sack of
flour, requires muscles to contract to overcome resistance.
Muscles that regularly overcome resistance get stronger. Without
periodic forays into overcoming resistance, muscles lose their
tone. That's why it is so important in our technological age to
make sure our muscles are allowed to do the contracting and
stretching they were designed to do. When we fall into our
technology trap of making life easier, we are more apt to lose
muscle tone and strength. Again, it's the old "use it or lose it"
syndrome. And "use it" means more than just keeping muscles
stress-tense from emotions.

Emotions can keep muscles tense and ready to go. And that's
good as long as the tense part is relatively short and is quickly
followed by the go part.

When you stand up, your back muscles are taut enough to
keep body upright against the pull of gravity. When you are lying
down, your muscles should relax. If a muscle is as taut when
you're lying down as it is when you're standing up, there's
nothing wrong with the muscle. It's ready to go into action. But
if the action doesn't follow and the tenseness remains, the muscle
is doing a perfect thing at an inappropriate time. After a while, it
gets tired.

WELLNESS PRINCIPLE: Ill-timed responses may
cause chronic backaches.

To re-time ill-timed responses, the Red or Yellow need to
provide updated information for the Green to respond to. With

updated information, the Green can reinstate normal resting muscle tone. That's retiming, or reintegration of neuromuscular communication. Reintegrating neuromuscular communication is the solution to ill-timed muscle responses. Constant negativity from the Red and residual tension from Yellow override can keep muscles slightly contracted and limit how much further they can contract. The object is to coordinate responses with current conditions. In the process, the muscles become more elastic and more moveable. Improved timing allows maximum relaxation which, in turn, allows for more contraction.

Adding a mental exercise to the Morter March can provide an opportunity that may help coordinate neuromuscular responses from Yellow override with current conditions.

As you stretch through the Morter March and hold your breath, allow your mind to focus on the first problem in your life that pops into your thoughts. It may be a situation you are currently dealing with, or it may be an incident in the past. You probably won't need to work at finding a negative thought on which to focus. When you think about things you wish hadn't happened or had turned out differently as you do the Morter March, the physical and mental are coordinated. These coordinated exercises can update the physiological responses attached to memories of the negative incident.

For the first week, each time you do the Morter March, allow thoughts of a particular negative experience to be the center of your attention. The same experience may or may not pop into your mind each time. Most of us have a nearly unlimited cache of negative memories available.

The second week, follow the same exercise routine. However this time, think of things about which you are passionate. These passions may include people, things or experiences you love more than anything, activities, favorite projects, causes, vacation plans, an impending wedding or birth, or whatever excites you positively and joyously.

Since I have been emphasizing the connection between

negative thoughts and Yellow override, you may wonder what thinking lovely wonderful thoughts has to do with retiming neuromuscular coordination.

My clinical experience demonstrates that, very often, patients' physiology responds dramatically when they think about subjects that give them extreme pleasure. We can become as excited and "stressed" physiologically by positive experiences as we can by negative experiences. The purpose of concentrating on positives during the Morter March is to retime physiological patterns, not to dilute the enjoyment of the thoughts.

After the two-week cycle of concentrating on negatives for the first week and positives for the second week, as you do the Morter March, allow your thoughts to focus on whatever is paramount in your mind at the time. Remember, the Morter March can not only stretch muscles and retime muscle responses, it can help to neutralize some of the effects of Yellow override.

Keep in mind that the Morter March stretching and retiming exercise isn't designed as a body-building exercise. It's a health-enhancing exercise. It's a bit of resistance to retone muscles, and an opportunity for retiming to update that tone.

WELLNESS PRINCIPLE: Retoning builds strength; retiming improves flexibility.

The Morter March is easy to do. It provides major muscles and joints a full range of motion. It retones muscles and retimes mind-body communication. It takes only about ten minutes a day. It's non-competitive. And it doesn't require membership fees or expensive equipment. So is that the only health-enhancing exercise you need?

Not necessarily.

An exercise program should be fun. If it isn't, many people won't stay with it. There are those who are highly disciplined and diligently exercise regularly whether it is enjoyable or not.

However, most of them are motivated by the returns they get despite the drudgery. Those who exercise for rehabilitation are a good example. There's strong motivation to exercise to help restore the use of a severely injured arm, leg, or back. But once the goal has been met, the motivation to continue may disappear.

Most exercise that increases the heart rate, improves flexibility, tones muscles, and generally energizes you can enhance your health. The type of exercise best for you depends on your own physical circumstances. So, let's look at how some of the more popular forms of exercise fit into the health-enhancing picture.

A GOOD SPORT

You may have noticed that recreational sports come in different types: vigorous or leisurely, contact or non-contact, outdoor or indoor, equipment intensive or equipment free, and so forth. Despite these differences, all sports involve individuals performing alone, or two or more individuals performing as a team. Team sports are essentially games and competitions; solo sports are essentially personal challenges.

Team sports are usually games in the sense that there is a winner and loser. We "play" games with other people: tennis, soccer, football, baseball, basketball, and the like.

Solo sports, on the other hand, are essentially an individual against himself or herself. Weight lifting, swimming, skiing, gymnastics, track and field events, auto racing, ice skating, and in-line skating are examples of solo sports. Although competition is often introduced into individual sports and individuals are gathered together as a team, they are essentially activities in which participants try to improve their personal best.

WELLNESS PRINCIPLE: Team sports are work-together sports; solo sports focus on individual performance.

The common denominator among all sports is that they combine fun, recreation, and a challenge. Yet these three ingredients are strictly subjective. For one person, basketball may rank high in all three. For another, it may score a minus in all three. Racing a high-performance car at barely sub-sonic speeds in the midst of a pack of similarly paced cars around a specially designed track may be a little bit of heaven for one person. His or her sibling may find just as much stimulation and thrill in the distinctly personal challenge of improving a personal best in weight-lifting.

Individual physical ability and personality play a large part in our selection of recreational exercise and what we consider fun. Intense competition may be stimulating for one person, but high level stress for another.

Most games and sports operate under rules. Strategies for winning are worked out within those rules. Consequently most sports have a strategic element as well as a physical element. And many people find that the mental activity associated with sports enhances the stimulation and satisfaction of the physical. Others prefer to put strenuous thinking on the back burner during physical activities.

What does all of this team and solo sport, fun, challenge, and personality business have to do with contralateral, mind-body integrating, muscle-toning, cardiovascular enhancing exercise?

It illustrates that there is no universally perfect exercise activity. The best exercise for you is that exercise that fits your personality. Even that most basic of all exercise — walking — may not be the most suitable long-term program for your personality. Walking doesn't pit your athletic skills and endurance against someone else. Although contralateral walking is definitely a boon to your whole-body condition, it may not satisfy your need for vigorous mental activity combined with vigorous physical activity.

WELLNESS PRINCIPLE: There is no one-size-fits-all

exercise.

The moral of all of this is that different sports and exercises offer different benefits. So let's look at a few popular forms of sports and exercises to see some of the pros and cons and how they fit our criteria of improving cardiovascular systems, muscle flexibility and tone, and mind-body communication.

Walking

Best overall exercise when movement is contralateral. A thirty-minute walk that combines ten-minute segments of slow-fast-slow offers aerobic and anaerobic benefits. Tones muscles, improves cardiorespiratory efficiency, and integrates mind-body communication. Walking can go on indefinitely. In the process, glucose goes from liver into blood, into muscle cell, into mitochondria and generates energy as rapidly as needed. Walking on a treadmill provides physical benefits, however, walking outdoors in natural surroundings can enhance the physical with fresh air for the body and the beauties of nature for the psyche.

Rhythmic Aerobics

Good contralateral movement for neuromuscular integration. Increases metabolism, cardiorespiratory rate, improves muscle tone. Over time, may improve bone density. Puts stress on joints. Non-competitive. Satisfying to those who prefer to compete against themselves. May be "boring" to those inclined toward team sports.

Water Aerobics

Good exercise especially for those with joint pain as long as water is warmed to at least 84° F. Offers the same benefits as rhythmic aerobics without the stress of weight on joints.

Swimming

Freestyle and backstroke are contralateral movements that offer the greatest whole body benefits. To provide optimal contralateral action during free-style stroke, breathing should be both to right and left sides during the swim (but don't try to squeeze in turns to both sides during one stroke). The four racing strokes — free-style, back-stroke, butterfly, and breast-stroke — give the aerobic system a good workout. The side-stroke is much more leisurely, but it isn't contralateral movement. In general, swimming is good, clean fun.

Tennis and Other Racquet Games
Combines aerobic and anaerobic benefits. Since the stroke used in tennis and other racquet games is essentially one-handed, much of the movement is not contralateral. To enhance the neuromuscular benefits of "one-sided" games, begin and end the session with a five-minute Morter March.

Jogging or Running
Aerobic, contralateral benefits. Put stress on feet, ankles, knees, and hips. Let your body rather than your conscious mind determine the distance and speed. Over-stressing muscles and joints can lead to injury. Running puts muscles into oxygen deficit, so muscles must rely on anaerobic processes to supply energy from carbohydrates. This can lead to lactic acid burn.

Baseball and Softball
Baseball and softball are more fun than they are aerobic exercise. Short bursts of intense exertion punctuate long periods of minimal physical activity. However, both games require physical coordination and skill, and they offer a competitive component that adds emotional excitement.

Cycling
Riding stationary exercise cycles and mobile bicycles provides aerobic benefits. Cycles are driven by leg power with the upper body riding along. Stationary exercise bikes with handlebars that

move along with the pedals allow for contralateral movement if the rider pushes the handle bars rather than pulls them. The bikes are designed so that one handle bar moves back as the leg on that side pushes down. Consequently, pulling the handlebar with one hand while pushing with the leg on the same side misses the benefits of contralateral movement. In conventional cycling, a limited number of muscles work at a high level of intensity which produces lactic acid.[48]

Cross-Country Skiing
Cross-country skiing, whether on a machine or on snow, uses many muscles. It is aerobic exercise with contralateral movement.

Golf
Golf, as played until the invention of the riding golf cart, is aerobic exercise with the added enjoyments of attractive natural surroundings and fresh air. Since the golf swing itself takes about 2 seconds of anaerobic power activity, when the player rides a motorized golf cart, most of the potential physical benefits of the game are lost. However, when the course is walked, golf is a whole-body enhancing aerobic, contralateral exercise.

Weight Training
Weight training is no longer just a "macho guy thing." Many women, and many older men and women, use weight training to tone muscles and build strength at home or at commercial fitness centers. Weight training is resistance training. It can increase flexibility, build strength of muscles, and improve bone density. Weight training can be short bursts of anaerobic exercise or aerobic exercise of longer periods of sustained movement against a resisting apparatus. It can enhance performance of both day-to-day and athletic activities.

DO SOMETHING!

No matter what your preference in exercise, you'll benefit only by doing it. Just thinking about exercising isn't enough.

There's no guarantee that exercising regularly will lengthen you life. But it may make your stay here in the land of the living more pleasant. Exercise is an energy user and an energy producer. You can demonstrate this for yourself the next time you wonder why you are so tired even though you haven't done much in the way of physical activity. Instead of slumping down in front of the TV, move — run in place, do pushups, do the Morter March. Do something physical to get your heart beating a little faster, your breathing a little deeper, and your blood coursing instead of dribbling through your veins. As internal activity increases, energy is renewed. You'll feel more less tired.

WELLNESS PRINCIPLE: Regularly push your body beyond sluggish.

Keep in mind that exercise is only one of the six essentials that determine how your body is functioning. Exercise stimulates production of physiologic acid. Consequently, exercise can push an overly acid body beyond the limits of its ability to compensate. So make sure your diet provides enough neutralizing minerals from vegetables and fruits for your body to handle the acid residue of dietary protein. A combination of body-friendly diet and regular exercise can help to overcome deficiencies in other areas of the six essentials, such as breathing, which we will talk about next.

CHAPTER 11

BREATHING IS NOT AN OPTION

BREATH-TAKING CHOICES

Breathing is a handy process. It's a natural talent. No training necessary. But it accomplishes much. It disposes of waste, adjusts metabolism, supplies a basic ingredient for energy, and is behind every word you speak. And as we have seen, controlled breathing combined with exercise can affect physiological timing.

Breathing is so essential that the idea of making breathing choices may seem a little far-fetched. We need oxygen to live, and while we're alive, we breathe. It's not an optional activity. And nature has provided enough oxygen for everyone.

> WELLNESS PRINCIPLE: Breathing is a built-in
> talent; stocking up on the
> "Big O" isn't necessary.

Breathing is one part of whole-body physiology. We won't discuss respiratory abnormalities or respiratory diseases. Breathing disorders should be handled by your doctor. We're talking here about whole-body health. Our purpose here is to air some choices you have when it comes to breathing.

The most obvious choice is whether or not to smoke cigarettes. That's a simple yes or no choice. The health hazards of cigarette smoking are well-known and well-publicized. So I'll add only one point rarely mentioned in the campaign against smoking.

Cigarettes have been termed drug delivery systems. A seldom-mentioned element is that when the smoker inhales cigarette smoke, all of ingredients in the smoke are delivered undiluted directly to the lungs. There is no filtering or screening process. The ingredients in the smoke are absorbed by the blood. The body has no opportunity or mechanism to counteract or neutralize the effects of the nicotine and other impurities before they are delivered directly to the blood. Nicotine is a poison. As one medical dictionary describes it, "Nicotine is one of the most toxic and addicting of all poisons."[49] So taking a drag on a cigarette and inhaling is an act of self-poisoning. Doesn't make much sense does it?

WELLNESS PRINCIPLE: Don't let your health go up
                                       in smoke.

While smoking is a yes or no choice, we make other choices in life that affect the quality of the air we breathe. Two of those choices are where we live and where we work. Locations and jobs that offer clean fresh air are ideal. But ideal locations combined with ideal jobs are few and growing fewer. Many of us live and breathe in a fog of air pollution. Automobile exhaust and industrial or agricultural pollutants are facts of life in many areas of the country. Yet these areas are where jobs are to be found. So, generally, there's considerably more involved than a simple "I will" or "I won't" in making choices of where you live and work. Circumstances, opportunities, and economics often dictate location and occupation.

You might live in a smog saturated city and work in a chemical-intensive environment. This is definitely an unfavorable combination. The ideal solution is to move and get a different job. But practicality wins out. You may not be able to change your location, and your expertise may be specific to a type of job that is prone to pollution. So moving or changing jobs may not be the most practical solution.

The next best solution is to keep your internal environment as healthy as possible to give your body a fighting chance to withstand your external environmental circumstances. And you can keep your internal environment in peak condition when you make sure your diet, rest, exercise, and thought choices are the best they can be. That way, even if you live and work in an atmospherically-challenged location, your superbly designed body has a better chance of handling the situation with fewer negative consequences.

WELLNESS PRINCIPLE: A favorable internal environment is the best defense
against an unfavorable
external environment.

Another breathing choice may not seem like a choice at all. It's about allowing yourself room to breathe.

Your lungs are protected by your rib cage. Your lungs expand in two ways: they lengthen or shorten according to the downward or upward movement of the diaphragm, and; they increase or decrease in diameter according to the elevation of the ribs. You can easily demonstrate these two movements.

First, put your fingers on your diaphragm just below your sternum (breastbone) and your thumb on your ribs at the side. Breathe normally — no big breath. Feel the up and down movement of the diaphragm with your fingers. But there's little, if any, movement of your ribs. Now, with your hand in the same position, take a deep breath. You should be able to feel your rib cage move. Actually, the ribs move upward. At rest, the ribs are slanted slightly downward. When you take a deep breath, the rib cage is elevated — the ribs project forward rather than downward.

That's an interesting bit of trivia. But so what?

It's a posture thing.

If you walk around with your chest caved in, the movement of your diaphragm is restricted. That restricts the movement of your lungs.

We were designed with lungs that have the capacity to serve our needs. We weren't equipped with more lung tissue than we need.. When you are resting your body doesn't need as much oxygen as when you are exercising. So you don't breathe as deeply when resting as when exercising. However, walking about isn't resting. When lung movement is restricted by poor posture, physiology can be affected. Breathing is more than an idle pastime. Cells need oxygen to function. Breathing takes in oxygen that goes to cells, and it eliminates carbon dioxide from the body. The straighter you stand, the better your lungs can do their job.

> WELLNESS PRINCIPLE: Stand up for your right to breathe well.

A DISCREET WASTE DISPOSAL SYSTEM

Breathing is a subconscious Green function. You don't need to learn how. And you don't need to think about how your body handles the breath after it goes in. Your subconscious takes care of the whole process. It handles the actual in and out process, it handles the substances you breathe in, and it handles the elimination of materials that need to be expelled.

> WELLNESS PRINCIPLE: Breathing is nothing to be sneezed at.

What's the main purpose of breathing?

Silly question. Everyone knows the purpose is to supply the body with oxygen. And everyone knows we need oxygen to live.

But there's more to it than that.

We not only breathe in, we breathe out. Exhaling is just as productive as inhaling. Inhaling brings in oxygen (among other elements and molecules). Exhaling removes waste materials, especially acid generated by cells.

The main purpose of breathing is to keep body fluids in the best condition possible. Breathing maintains the best survival-blend possible of oxygen, carbon dioxide and hydrogen ions in body fluids.[50] Cells work best in a slightly alkaline environment. Breathing is a major part of your internal environmental control.

We talked earlier about the acid factor in the body — acid from acid ash-producing foods and acid from cellular function. Dietary acid from protein foods is eliminated through the digestive tract. Acid produced by cells in their normal course of business is gathered in the blood stream, sent through the lungs, and exhaled as carbon dioxide and water. In fact, a hundred times more acid is eliminated in the form of carbon dioxide and water than any other acid eliminated from the body.[51] It's an ingenious acid management system. If we could manage our personal, national, and global resources and capabilities as well as the body manages its resources and capabilities, we'd all be able to breathe a lot easier.

WELLNESS PRINCIPLE: The body is the original
efficiency expert.

The job of acid removal might appear to be a completely chemical process. Actually, acid removal is a survival function from way back. It begins in the primitive brain. That's the part that has been around the longest. Part of your Green. And your Green works whether you do or not.

The medulla oblongata and pons are parts of your lower brain. They look rather like bulbous extensions of the spinal cord. These small, lumpy-looking masses of nerve tissue have areas that are highly sensitive to changes in carbon dioxide or hydrogen ion concentrations in the blood. And excess carbon dioxide and hydrogen ions in the blood mean acidosis. We know that's not good. When these sensitive areas of the brain detect an increase in physiological acid, they signal the respiratory centers. The respiratory centers handle the situation by increasing the respiratory rhythm.[52] You breathe faster. Faster breathing, more acid elimination. Great system!

> WELLNESS PRINCIPLE: Breathing is your built-in central "vacuum" system.

You breathe faster and deeper when you exercise because your metabolic processes work faster when you exercise. Everything speeds up. Cells work faster and produce more acid. Muscles work harder and produce more acid. The pH in both tissue and tissue blood can drop as much as 0.5.[53] And if blood must stay between pH 7.35 and 7.45, a 0.5 drop in pH means it's crisis time. So breathing hard when you exercise can be a life saver.

OK, if the body is so smart yet it generates acid that must be eliminated, one might think the body would be designed to function without generating acid.

Perhaps in another cosmos, waste-free energy production might be possible. But in our world, materials are *exchanged* for energy, not eliminated. As with all living animals and plants, the body continually exchanges materials and energy.[54] In the body, this energy exchange is called metabolism.

METABOLIZE TO ENERGIZE
You may have heard people complain or brag about their metabolism. "I can't lose weight because my metabolism is slow." Or, "I have all this energy because my metabolism is so fast." But what is metabolism?

Metabolism is the body's combined processes that make internal energy available.[55] Metabolism is the chemical processes that allow cells to continue to live.[56] So you can see that it's in your best interest to treat your body in ways that promote the most effective metabolism. The more efficient your metabolism the more energy you have. The more energy you have, the better your whole body functions, the better you feel, and the more you can do. And that's the purpose of making the best choices possible in the six essentials.

> WELLNESS PRINCIPLE: Metabolism is your
>   energizer.

We get our energy from the food we eat. The substances in food are broken down in the body and converted to energy. It's all done at the molecular level. The cereal you have for breakfast and the hamburger you have for lunch are in reality a collection of molecules. Each of us is a collection of molecules. That's a humbling thought. However, this view of yourself and everyone else gives new meaning to the concept "all men are created equal." And when you're rooting for your home team, you're really saying "My favorite molecule groups can beat your favorite molecule groups."

You can see that molecules and metabolism are important to health and exercise.

We get energy from food when it is broken down. Food is fuel ready to be converted to energy by chemical reactions. That's the job of your cells: make energy in foods available for physiological processes. Oxygen is needed for much of this energy conversion. Carbohydrates, fats, and proteins can be oxidized in cells.

Oxidation is the process of combining with oxygen. In the process, large amounts of energy are released. Outside the body, you get a similar effect by burning the food with pure oxygen. The difference is that outside the body the energy released is in the form of heat. Inside the body, the energy released by oxidation is used for muscle movement and other functions. Oxygen is needed in both processes. And a residual ash is left from both processes. Another example of oxidation is the old, rusty nail. The rust is a result of a much slower oxidation process than either burning or physiological oxidation. But in the process, energy is released and a residual "ash" is left.

> WELLNESS PRINCIPLE: Metabolism and energy are oxygen-dependent.

It will come as no surprise to you that both energy and ash are pertinent to our topics of health and exercise. So, let's tie together a few of the concepts we've discussed in this book.

METABOLIC ENERGY

In chapter 6 of this book, we talked about ATP — adenosine triphosphate. ATP is made in the mitochondria — the power-house of cells. In the mitochondria, nutrients from food are combined with oxygen to form ATP. ATP is the "fuel" cells use to perform physiological functions. It's made from carbohydrates. We get carbohydrates when we eat plant materials — grapes, wheat, broccoli, pineapple, oats, carrots, rice, potatoes, and the like. The energy from about 99% of all the carbohydrates used by the body is used to form ATP.[57] And nearly all physiological functions that require energy get that energy from ATP or a similar high energy compound.[58]

Just about all of the of carbohydrates you eat and digest end up as glucose.[59] "Glucose" is the sophisticated scientific term for the sugar "dextrose" — the sugar in corn syrup and honey. Glucose is more than just a type of sugar. It comes mainly from digesting starches. And here's another bit of dinner table trivia: the word "glucose" comes from the Greek word for "sweet" referring to new wine.[60]

> WELLNESS PRINCIPLE: Glucose is the most impor-
> tant carbohydrate in body metabolism.

Glucose metabolism changes chemical energy from food to mechanical energy or heat.[61] About 90% of all ATP is formed by glucose metabolism.[62] Glucose is absorbed from the intestines by the blood, processed through other organs such as the liver, and ends up in the cells.[63] Once absorbed by the cells, the glucose can either be used immediately to release energy, or it can be stored.[64] If the glucose isn't needed immediately for energy, it is stored either as glycogen or fat. Cells store enough glycogen to meet their needs for 12 to 24 hours. The rest can end up in fat cells.[65]

WELLNESS PRINCIPLE: Glycogen is a use-as-energy
or store-as-fat product.

The body has several intricate processes for changing food energy into ATP and usable energy. The principle function of these processes is to transform the glucose from food into a form that can be combined with oxygen. Ninety percent of ATP is formed by further-processing glucose to make hydrogen atoms available in forms that can be used in oxidation.[66] Oxidation is the process of combining a substance with oxygen. It's an aerobic process — aerobic means "in the presence of oxygen."

Aerobic exercises are "in" these days. During aerobic exercise, energy is supplied by the oxygen that is breathed in.[67] To keep up hard physical exercise, you need to breathe in lots of oxygen. And in the process of this exercising and breathing, the heart pumps harder and faster. More oxygen-filled blood is delivered to the cells, and more ATP can be manufactured to keep muscles contracting and relaxing on cue. When you run, chop wood, shovel snow, or otherwise work your muscles for long periods, you huff and puff. You aren't just refilling your lungs, you're refueling your cells.

WELLNESS PRINCIPLE: Huffing and puffing is a
refueling process for long-

term exertion.

Your body is not a shoddy, low-tech, low-budget product. It has backup systems. And it has backup systems to backup systems. If you should stop breathing for a minute or so, you can survive and your muscles can still respond. And in your daily activities, you don't immediately start to breathe harder the moment you begin to do something strenuous. If you are in reasonably good shape, you can run across the street or lift a bag of groceries and your breathing rate changes very little. Muscle fuel for these short-term lapses in oxygen supply or bursts of energy come from related, but different, systems. They don't require an immediate surge of oxygen to get you going.

Cell energy can be generated anaerobically. Anaerobic — without oxygen. Anaerobic glycolysis is the process in the cells of converting glucose to ATP and energy without using oxygen. ATP can form in muscle cells without new oxygen for short periods. The process is called anaerobic glycolysis. Anaerobic systems are great life-saving devices and useful for "quick energy." Anaerobic processes help you out for short energy bursts like a 100-yard dash, weight lifting, and jumping. But when you run the Boston marathon or simply jog, your aerobic system is the energy producer.

Keep in mind that the main purpose of cellular activity is survival. To survive, cells must produce energy. Glucose is the principal fuel for cells. Much of the activity of cells is directed toward converting glucose to glycogen which eventually is used for energy. But as with most fuels, glucose energy production leaves by-products.

When plenty of oxygen is available to help in the glucose conversion process (aerobic glycolysis), one of the main by-products is carbon dioxide. Your body gets rid of excess carbon dioxide when you breathe. Anaerobic glycolysis, on the other hand, brings about the production of lactic acid in muscles. Lactic acid is a specific mixture of carbon, hydrogen, and oxygen. Lactic acid is well-known as an ingredient in milk and milk products. And for another piece of trivia, it's also formed in sauerkraut, and certain types of pickles. But of more importance here, lactic acid is formed by muscular activity.[68] The lactic acid is a by-product of turning glucose into energy. Cells get energy from the glycogen-lactic acid boost for about 30 or 40 seconds. This energy system contributes fuel to muscles to take you through strenuous, longer-than-a-sprint events such as 100-meter swim races.[69]

> WELLNESS PRINCIPLE: Muscles can form their own
> energy-producers for short-
> term work.

But when you run for an hour or so, lactic acid builds up in the muscles. Lactic acid build-up in muscles causes extreme fatigue. To recover, excess lactic acid must be eliminated from the body. About an hour is needed for the body to eliminate large amounts of lactic acid that has been produced and fully recover.[70] The lactic acid is broken down and "neutralized," and the acid in the form of carbon dioxide is eliminated through the lungs.[71] Once again we have a situation of surviving excess.

So we have anaerobic energy release systems that fuel muscles for up to 40 seconds, and we have aerobic energy release to handle vigorous activity for the long-haul. Weight lifting and other anaerobic exercises done on a regular basis help to strengthen muscles. And that's good for people of every age. However, anaerobic exercises don't have as much effect on the cardiovascular system as aerobic exercises.

Aerobic exercises, such as jogging and lap-swimming, have a whole-body effect. They help tone muscles and strengthen the built-in heart-lung machine. Aerobic exercises require a lot of oxygen. And when oxygen is used to get energy from ATP, muscles have about ten times more energy available than they get from anaerobic systems.

We hear a great deal about aerobic exercises improving the cardiovascular system. What that means is that with exercise, the heart and blood vessels can deliver more oxygen to the muscles. And it also improves the ability of muscle fibers to use the oxygen they get.[72]

WELLNESS PRINCIPLE: Breathing feeds muscles.

Keep in mind that this is not a physiology text. The explanations of how muscles are energized are greatly simplified overviews of extremely complex internal processes. The purpose here is to illustrate the connection between breathing and strenuous (or any) exercise. The point is that when you exercise, anaerobic activity starts you out. It's short-term. Aerobic activity that uses energy from food joins in later to keep you going. It's long-term.

If you exercise regularly, you may have noticed that when you begin your workout you don't get out of breath right away. Anaerobic processes are supplying energy to your muscles. But after a few minutes, you begin to work harder to take in more air. If you continue your workout, gradually you aren't as "winded" as you were. You get your "second wind." That's the aerobic process when oxygen becomes available to help burn fuel.[73]

Acid is produced in the cells by both aerobic and anaerobic exercise. And if you are going to keep going, your body needs to change food into energy, and it needs to get rid of the acid generated when cells function using the energy.

WELLNESS PRINCIPLE: Exercise, like some foods, is
                     an acid-producer.

Your body isn't stupid. It wasn't designed to produce a potentially dangerous by-product, such as acid, without having a method of getting rid of it. Every time you exhale, you are removing cell-generated acid from your body.

As a reminder, cell-generated acid is eliminated through the lungs when you exhale, but dietary acid from acid ash foods must be neutralized and eliminated through the digestive tract. An important difference. You can't "blow-off" acid from acid ash foods. Acid from exercise is in the body only a short time. Acid from acid ash foods hangs around a lot longer. Which brings us back to diet and the pH level of the body.

EXERCISE AND pH
The body was designed to be slightly alkaline, but excess dietary protein over a long period can lead to "acid buildup." And since most of us eat much more protein than our bodies need, most of us are more acid than we were designed to be.

The ideal blood pH is between 7.35 and 7.45. That's slightly alkaline. But how can you know how your particular pH level stacks up against the ideal? As a quick indicator of the acid level of your internal environment, try this short "Breath Test" exercise. You'll need a watch or clock with a second hand.

Remember, this exercise is a general indicator; it's not a diagnostic tool. Only your doctor can diagnose a disease and put a name on it.

The Breath Test
Lie down quietly for a few minutes. Relax. Take a couple of deep breaths. Relax. Now, take a deep breath and hold it. Time yourself to see how long you can hold your breath without exhaling. That means no "leaking." You won't learn anything if you let the air seep quietly out of your lungs. The objective is to see how long you can hold your breath before you MUST exhale and take another breath.

Breath-holding tolerance is influenced by many physiological factors, such as the ammonia backup system for neutralizing acid. The breath-holding test is an acid indicator principally for those who are "reasonably healthy" and not on a regular regime of medication.

The ability to hold your breath for at least one minute may indicate that your body has managed to keep your acid level under control. Even so, your internal environment may be more acidic than it was designed to be. However, apparently, your blood can still carry enough oxygen for your body to sustain itself for a minute during complete oxygen deprivation. As a general rule, the longer you can hold your breath, the less acid your body; the shorter period of time you can hold your breath, the more acid your body. I have some patients who can hold their breath for a minute and a half or longer. Other patients can't hold it at all. They take a deep breath and seem to "explode" immediately in search of more air.

If you can't hold your breath for about a minute, your body may be overly acid from excess dietary protein.

You can see the relationships among cell metabolism, holding your breath, and an acid interior. Cells use oxygen when they function. You get oxygen when you breathe in, and eliminate acid when you breathe out. If your internal environment is overly acid, your infinite intelligence will insist on eliminating exhalable acid as quickly as possible. Eliminating dietary acid takes longer than eliminating cellular acid. So the acid that can go out through your lungs must go as quickly as possible. You can't do long-term breath-holding when your body must contend with a lot of acid. And acid generated by strenuous exercise may overload physiological neutralizing systems. So if you can't hold your breath for about a minute, you may need to improve your diet before you exercise strenuously.

MORE ABOUT BREATH-HOLDING

Breathing is a survival process. Basic survival processes are controlled by your Green subconscious. On the list of survival priorities, breathing ranks right up at the top along with other Green-directed functions — pumping heart, circulating blood, and control of physiology. If any of these Green functions stops completely, the body doesn't have much of a future. So breathing is a top priority of the body.

The difference between breathing and the other three priorities is that breathing is not only a Green function, you have some Red conscious control over it. Of course, if you devote your conscious activity to controlling breathing, you won't have much time to think about anything else. Nonetheless, you have more Red control over the rate and depth of your breathing than you have over your heart rate, blood circulation, and internal information network. You may be able to affect those, but you can't control them. Breathing is in a class by itself. You can use this conscious control to help you relax. Not only that, you can use it to help re-time your internal communication systems.

> WELLNESS PRINCIPLE: Red intent can override Green breathing — for short periods.

When you hold your breath, you consciously override subconscious control of breathing. But breathing is a survival priority. Hold your breath and you "short circuit" one of the body's survival processes. Not only is the oxygen supply cut off, but respiratory acid can't be eliminated. And acid accumulation is a tremendous threat to the body. So breathing becomes not just one of the top priorities, it becomes THE top priority. There's an internal crisis brewing. So, what does the body do?

At first it tenses to handle the threat. Then, it relaxes.

It relaxes to slow down internal processes that consume oxygen and produce acid. Tense muscles do both — consume oxygen and produce acid. When oxygen is in short supply, your body ignores signals from your Yellow non-conscious that have been keeping it ready to run or fight. Energy is no longer wasted on unnecessary internal activities.

You may have noticed the muscle-relaxing response when you did the Breath Test to see how long you could go without breathing. At first you were prepared for the process that your conscious mind knew might be uncomfortable. Then, just before you had to breathe, you may have noticed a feeling of relaxation. Muscles relaxed. The feeling might be described as "melting" into the bed, floor, or whatever you were lying on.

WELLNESS PRINCIPLE: Holding your breath is a
                      relaxing experience —
                      eventually.

Now, why would your body relax at such a dangerous time? To conserve life-sustaining resources. It's a re-timing process. The body is no longer wasting energy on trying to cope with lesser threats of Uncle George or rebellious children or the IRS. Your Green shuts down unnecessary activity. All of those mental threats that keep the body on guard fade when the primary threat to survival is oxygen deprivation and acid accumulation.

When your body is deprived of oxygen, tense muscles are unnecessary. Muscles need oxygen to contract. When you hold your breath, the body will find any source of available oxygen. The oxygen that would have gone to muscles to keep them tense is available to keep the cells alive.

Although muscles use a lot of oxygen, your brain is the major oxygen consumer. It uses more oxygen than any other organ. Without oxygen, brain cells can't function. And different areas of the brain control particular organs. So when the oxygen supply is threatened, even parts of the brain that aren't contributing to keeping you alive slow down to conserve oxygen. Consequently, the organs controlled by those brain areas slow down also. The principal threat is to survival as a whole, not survival of parts. The body's response is directed toward survival of the whole. If that means slowing organic processes, so be it. Survival is the only consideration.

WELLNESS PRINCIPLE: Holding your breath puts a
                      different   perspective   on

individual threats.

Holding your breath shifts survival priorities slowly, at first. Then after several seconds, the crisis builds and the greatest stress is the need to breathe. And as the need increases, changes take place not only in organs but in internal communication between brain and organs. Your internal communication is re-timed.

We might think of internal timing and rhythms as being like the timing and rhythm of a pendulum clock. As the pendulum swings along smoothly, the systems of clock function smoothly and in time. And it does this until interference comes along. For the clock, interference may be a bump or something else that causes asynchronous fluctuations. The timing and rhythm are out of synch. For the body, the interference may be coming from Yellow override, but timing and rhythms still get out of synch. To get the clock rhythm and timing back in synch, you stop the pendulum, give it a nudge, and its rhythms and timing are again coordinated. In the body, when you intentionally stop breathing until breathing becomes an absolute necessity, the brain shuts down activities and systems that are unnecessary to immediate survival. These activities and systems are then nudged back into energy-conserving synchronized timing. When the breathless crisis is over, the body can maintain the re-timed rhythm. At least it can maintain it until the next crisis, which will probably come from thoughts.

WELLNESS PRINCIPLE: In   health,   timing   is
                              everything.

As long as you are alive, you will breathe. And your survival oriented Green will see to it that you do. If the conscious breath-holding crisis were to go on too long, you would pass out — lose consciousness. Then your Green is really in command of everything. No Red interference, and no Yellow override while you're unconscious. Green does it all. And the first thing it does is to start you breathing again. However, I'm not suggesting that you try to hold your breath long enough to lose consciousness. Just long enough to shove Red and Yellow out of the way and let your Green handle your physiology without interference. When that happens, your muscles relax and your body is able to function most efficiently.

WELLNESS PRINCIPLE: A well-tuned body can use
more oxygen better.

When you combine holding your breath with contralateral exercise such as the Morter March, you give your body the greatest opportunity to re-time itself.

Breathing is just one of the six essentials for maintaining or improving health. Just as a refresher, the six essentials are: what you eat and what you drink, how you exercise, rest, and breathe, and how you think. All six of the essentials are interconnected. Each can affect the other. So let's look at how rest fits into not only your health picture but also your exercise program.

WELLNESS PRINCIPLE: The better your choices, the
better your health.

CHAPTER 12

. . . AND THE REST

TIME WELL INVESTED

Rest and sleep are essential. Your body needs both. Your brain needs both. Restful sleep gives your body time to convert food nutrients into fuel and to clean up its internal environment. Restful sleep allows muscles to relax and the body to focus on replenishing and repairing itself. From cells to systems, the body gears down and attends to internal needs while you sleep restfully. We might say that when the eyelids shut, the mind calms, and muscles relax, the body has hung out a "Temporarily Closed for Renovation" sign.

However, not everyone "rests" while they sleep. If you awaken in the morning as tired as when you went to bed, you may have slept, but you didn't rest. Your body couldn't replenish itself as efficiently as possible, and some muscles may not have rested at all.

During sleep, physiological activities slow, consciousness is diminished, and voluntary physical activity is absent.[74] You're not alert during sleep, but you can easily return to normal awareness — you can awaken. Your Red conscious mind idles, your Yellow memory hums along, and your Green subconscious is at full throttle taking care of the body's needs. In essence, while you sleep, your physiology is completely Green-driven.

Your Green is responding only to internal feedback information
from organs, muscles, and the like. Ideally, your Green is going
about its business without having to respond to signals from Red
and Yellow that indicate major or minor crises.

> WELLNESS PRINCIPLE: The best rest is Yellow
> absent, Green dominant.

By definition, rest is freedom from activity of both mind and
body. When you are resting but awake, your metabolism slows.
But it doesn't slow as much as it does while you are asleep.
During wakeful rest, your conscious Red continues to receive and
screen information from the outside world and to feed sensory
information to your Yellow and Green. You can slump into a
comfortable chair for a few minutes of physical rest between
chores or activities, but you are still awake, alert, thinking, and
receiving sensory stimuli. Muscles may be more relaxed than
they were when you were standing and active; however, your
Green is responding to Red and Yellow. So, in effect, you are
"resting" on the outside, while it's business as usual on the
inside. Whether you are awake or asleep, if your thoughts keep
churning, your body isn't truly resting.

> WELLNESS PRINCIPLE: Restless thoughts make for
> a restless body.

We have been taught that the purpose of rest is to refresh and
re-energize the body so we can get up and have another go at life.
Rest allows the body time to repair, rejuvenate, and renovate
itself. But that is just *one* purpose.

Another, perhaps more important, purpose is to allow the
body sufficient opportunity to re-time internal communications.
And that's one of the major themes of this book — your body
needs to be able to re-time itself. Re-timing is the refreshing
factor. When your body is well-timed, it is responding only to

sensory conditions of the moment — not to Yellow override. Your body is well-timed when it is responding to current events and emotions as opposed to memories of past events and emotions.

WELLNESS PRINCIPLE: In business, sports, and health, timing is everything.

Adequate rest is essential to good health. That's hardly a new concept. When we're sick, rest is high on the list of treatments. It's part of the standard formula promoted by health-directed special interest and commercial groups.

Rest is a natural process. The body demands it, and that demand will be met. We get tired; we rest. It's cyclical. We must rest frequently. Like the breathing essential, we don't always have absolute control over rest, but we usually do. We usually choose when and where we rest or sleep. But we can't stay awake indefinitely and we can't sleep indefinitely. And we can't work indefinitely without rest. The body won't allow it. If you push periods of wakefulness to extreme, you'll sleep whether you decide to or not.

Even insomniacs sleep sometime. We don't die from lack of sleep. Insomnia has never made the "Killer of the Year" list. Insomnia is defined as the inability to sleep, or spontaneously interrupted sleep. It is most frequently caused by anxiety or pain. Insomnia itself isn't a disease, although it may be a symptom of disease.[75] But no matter what you call it, lack of restful sleep can lower the body's resistance to disease.

Lack of restful sleep can also affect your ability to work efficiently and, more important, safely. Whether you're a student or astronaut, how well rested your body is affects how well, and how safely, you do your job. Fatigue may not be scientifically quantifiable, nevertheless, it can be a major factor in accidents and miscalculations.

For many, lack of rest or adequate sleep comes from self-inflicted time-pressures. We don't have time to take a vacation, "eat right," exercise, read a good book, smell the roses, or waste more than a few hours a night sleeping. Ben Franklin could have been describing our late twentieth century attitude when he wrote the now-familiar mottos, "Time is money," and "Do not squander time, for that's the stuff life is made of." But, resting and sleep are not time squanderers. They are essentials. An Irish proverb puts it best: "The beginning of health is sleep."

WELLNESS PRINCIPLE: Our bodies insist on rest.

So, how much sleep do we need?

SLEEP — HOW MUCH IS ENOUGH?
The traditional answer to the question of how much sleep we need is "eight hours." This eight-hour concept is so firmly ingrained that some people seem to feel their constitutional rights have been violated if they miss a part of their personal nightly allotment. Others seem to feel that they are guilty of "the deadly sin" of sloth if they exceed their allotted sack time.

The amount and quality of sleep *you need* each night depends on your stage of life and your overall health. And, the amount and quality of sleep *you get* during the night depends on the same things.

The small bodies of growing children need more sleep than do those of the fully-grown adults. Again, we have an example of the wisdom of design: not only do little people need to sleep a lot, their parents need for them to sleep a lot. And anyone who has been closely associated with rapidly growing teenagers is familiar with their capacity for sleep. Not only are their bodies still growing, but their hormonal systems are undergoing major transformations. Their bodies are in serious transition.

In addition to the growing generation, those who are ill need more rest and sleep than those who are healthy. Major body repair requires more restful "down time" than does regular body maintenance.

Not surprisingly, sleep researchers have found that younger people — twenty-something and younger — sleep more deeply and with fewer interruptions than older people. The body does much of its repair and reconstruction during deep sleep. As we age, our sleep becomes more fragmented. The over-65 group tends to wake several times each night — perhaps as many as a dozen times. And they descend less often into deep sleep.[76]

Yet, even with the fragmented sleep pattern that comes with age, the amount of dream time is reduced very little. Young, twenty-something sleepers dream for about two hours during the night; older, eighty-something sleepers log about an hour of dreaming. Dreaming is characterized by rapid eye movements during sleep. One researcher described rapid eye movement (REM) sleep as "a kind of psychological recuperation, as working out emotional issues." So, while we may get significantly less body-repairing deep sleep as we age, we hang on to "psychological recuperation" sleep.[77]

WELLNESS PRINCIPLE: Both body and mind benefit
                     from restful sleep.

About six hours of restful sleep each night *should* be adequate for most adults. In about six hours, a healthy body can tend to its maintenance, housekeeping, rebuilding, and restocking. Unfortunately, the bodies of "most people" in this country fall short of being truly healthy. They (the bodies) suffer from survival overload and nutrient deprivation brought on by combating the fallout from a steady diet of inappropriate choices. As a result, six hours may not be enough. Or, as with many of my patients, they can't put together six hours of uninterrupted sleep. If they get four or five hours at a stretch, they think they have done well.

WELLNESS PRINCIPLE: Sleep quantity and quality

depend on health; health
depends on making
appropriate choices.

Although we generally use the eight-hour mark as a guideline, you may not need that much, or you may need more.

Suppose, as a health-conscious person, you believe you need eight hours of sleep. But you have a tendency toward insomnia. You go to bed at 10:30 every night because you have to get up at 6:30 in the morning. That's eight hours, just as the doctor and custom order. But, instead of drifting off to sleep right a way, you lie awake, and frustrated, until midnight. Or, perhaps you go to sleep easily, but you come fully awake at 5 o'clock, and lie there until the alarm goes off at 6:30. Perhaps you aren't suffering from insomnia at all. Maybe your body is trying to tell you something. Maybe it is trying to tell you that you don't really need eight hours of sleep every night. Maybe your body does quite well with six-and-a-half hours of sleep each night. You'll get an idea of whether your sleep patterns are shortened because you're just too tied up to sleep restfully or because your particular body can tend to its resting, restoring, and re-energizing in less than eight hours. Try going to bed later or getting up when you wake up, instead of when "it's time."

Or, suppose you get your allotted eight hours of sleep through the 10:30 to 6:30 routine every night, but every morning when the alarm goes off at 6:30 you have to drag yourself to your feet and into the day. Maybe your body is telling you that the traditional eight hours just doesn't do the job for you. Try going to bed earlier, even if it means taking a few verbal barbs from family and friends. You will probably find that your days are more enjoyable, that you are more energetic, and that the early-to-bed jokes soon become stale.

WELLNESS PRINCIPLE: Sleep requirements are
personal — not dictated by

custom, habit, or peer
pressure.

The best way to determine just how much sleep your
particular body and mind need is to go to bed when you are
sleepy and wake up naturally. You may find that five or six hours
suits you just fine. Or you may find that your body leans toward
nine hours or so. Your job is to fit your active schedule to your
body's sleep schedule. You will know you have a perfect fit
when you don't need to "take something" to go to sleep, and you
don't need an alarm clock to awaken.

Now this business of "go to bed when you're sleepy and stay
there until you wake up" sounds ideal and all very well and good
for the independently wealthy or retired sets. But that may not be
at all practical for many who have a time clock to punch, an hour
or so commute each way to work, a family to attend to, shopping
to do, clothes to pick up at the cleaners, civic duties to perform,
and, in general, a full life and cluttered schedule. Sleep is often
the first thing to go to make room for obligations and
responsibilities. What do you do then?

This brings us back to choices.

Proper, adequate rest is one of the six essentials of health.
You have the choice of whether or not you allow time for your
body to relax and repair. However, the reasons for short-
changing the rest essential can also be behind short-changing
other essential choices. Exercise, proper diet, and especially
thoughts and attitudes can suffer when your schedule is over
packed. So not allowing yourself to get enough rest is often a
symptom of a larger problem. And the big problem is that your
life is controlling you — you aren't controlling your life.

If you can read this book, you are in a position to take control
of your life. You, and only you, can make the choices that are
best for your body and health. Choices that short-change one of
the six essentials occasionally probably won't alter your health
permanently. However, choices that consistently short-change
several of the six essentials may write your ticket to pain and ill-

health.

Sleep is a natural process. It serves a survival purpose of repair and rebuilding. The body knows how much sleep it needs. It doesn't need drugs to accomplish a natural process. If you need sedating pills to go to sleep and an alarm clock to wake up, you are disturbing a natural process by imposing Red decisions on a Green function.

> WELLNESS PRINCIPLE: Your body is the best judge
> of how much sleep you
> need.

FULL RANGE OF RELAXATION

Just as your body needs proper food to "refuel" and re-energize, it needs rest and relaxation to repair and re-time itself.

Rest is the counterweight of exercise and activity. Exercise strengthens muscles. Rest following exercise allows circulation in muscles to improve and lean muscle mass to be built. If one of your purposes in exercising is to build muscle and improve your physical appearance, (and what self-respecting "exercise nut" wouldn't want firm, well-developed muscles?), round-the-clock exercising won't get you where you want to go. Strenuous exercise breaks down muscle tissue. Rest allows tissue to repair and build up. Overexercising can actually reduce muscle mass.[78] This is why it's a good idea to schedule your exercise program in an every-other-day format. Work the muscles, then give them a chance to rebuild.

Muscles rest when they are relaxed. Rested muscles, and muscles that are capable of fully relaxing respond more efficiently when called into action.

For maximum movement and flexibility, muscles need to start movement from a relaxed state. When muscles start out partially tense, their range of motion is reduced. It's rather like the difference between a full swing of a baseball bat and a bunt. The full swing — full range of motion — is more powerful than the shortened — contracted — bunt movement.

Exercise is an opportunity for the musculoskeletal system to benefit from full range of motion movement. Rest is the opportunity for muscles to benefit from full range of relaxation. Muscles that are relaxed are more "elastic" and have a greater power potential.

WELLNESS PRINCIPLE: Full range of relaxation
allows full range of motion.

Just because we rest and sleep is no guarantee that our muscle groups are relaxed. Muscles that never rest can become very painful.

One of the greatest challenges to a chiropractor or other doctor is the patient who hobbles into the office with excruciating back pain, but no obvious cause. This patient is the fellow who got out of bed in the morning, bent over to tie his shoe or brush his teeth, and his back "went out." Not only was he in great pain, he couldn't straighten up. Yet he hadn't done anything out of the ordinary. He hadn't lifted a great weight improperly — neither shoe laces nor toothbrushes are overly heavy. He hadn't curled himself into a strange position — he had followed the same shoe-tieing and tooth-brushing routine every day. So what happened? Why did his back "go out"?

My clinical experience shows that his back didn't really go anyplace — his muscles were exhausted.

While he was sleeping, he wasn't resting. He was tense and his back muscles were contracted. Blood flow was restricted, metabolism increased, lactic acid built up, and muscle exhaustion set in. But he is totally unaware of the drama taking place in his back. So he gets up and gets dressed, or bends over to brush his teeth. In the process, he stretches the exhausted muscles beyond their current physiological limit. Wham! Muscle spasms send him to his knees in pain.

Millions of Americans suffer from "unexplained" back pain.

In all too many instances, the pain "just happened." It wasn't the result of an injury. The person didn't fall off a ladder or trip over a cat. The pain comes from muscle exhaustion even though the person had appeared to be getting enough sleep.

WELLNESS PRINCIPLE: Sleep is not always restful.

In general, while you are awake, your sympathetic nervous system is in charge of physiology. Muscles maintain waking muscle tone. You are ready to meet the many challenges and "threats" picked up by your sensory system. And during wakefulness, your Yellow is hard at work relating present sensations to memories of past similar situations. That's the way it should be. That's how we live. Calling on memories of past experiences to respond alertly for survival of conditions of the moment. But when the memories keep us in survival mode, neither body nor mind can rest. Neither body nor mind can work at maximum efficiency when required to function continuously for long periods without rest and sleep.

During restful sleep, your body switches its focus from survival sympathetic functions to restorative parasympathetic functions. Muscle tone decreases, blood pressure falls, pulse rate slows, and, if necessary, digestive activity increases. This is rest and repair time — resting homeostasis. Debris from the day's intake of food is gathered for elimination. Metabolism slows. Cells rejuvenate and reproduce. Wounds heal. The body is re-energized. And since life is energy, recharging your internal batteries can mean the difference between being lively and merely being alive. We need rejuvenating rest and sleep. No organ or system of the body — including the brain and central nervous system — can function full-tilt, full-time without rest.

REST IS A MIND THING
We ordinarily think of sleep as a cure for physical fatigue. And, indeed, it is. Yet, sleep benefits the central nervous system as

much as — if not more than — it benefits muscles.

After a hard day on a construction site, trekking ten miles as a letter carrier, working in the garden, or playing a couple sets of tennis, we can rest tired muscles and aching feet by sitting down and relaxing. And after a hard day at a desk or assembly line job, we can relieve stiff muscles by moving around. Changing position or patterns of activity can reduce muscle tension and re-energize body and mind.

A hard day at work can be physically taxing, mentally taxing, or both. A job, by definition, is a specific duty or function. And since most jobs involve specific functions, these functions are often repetitive. The repetition may not be physically performing exactly the same movements, but, rather, mentally focusing in the same area. The same areas of the brain are involved in carrying out the specific duties and functions. For example, a dentist may fill a tooth of one patient, put a crown on the tooth of another, treat a third for periodontal disease, and continue through the day analyzing and treating assorted dental conditions of assorted patients. Each patient poses a particular challenge and requires a specific treatment, but it's all dentistry. And it all requires thinking about how best to treat each patient. The dentist's mind is "working out of its dentistry areas" all day long. And after a full day of focused mental activity, fatigue sets in. It isn't so much that the muscles, tendons, and ligaments have been over stressed; it's the mind that is tired. The weary dentist is ready to go home and relax. But suppose just before the last patient arrives, a friend calls with an invitation to a quick set or two of tennis before the sun goes down.

All of a sudden, this tired dentist turns into an invigorated tennis player. Mental and physical fatigue vanish. The body hasn't rested at all, yet the center of activity in the brain has shifted.

WELLNESS PRINCIPLE: Fatigue often starts in the
brain.

The body doesn't truly rest as long as the mind is churning or emotions are boiling or simmering. Sitting down or otherwise changing patterns of physical activity can be a relief for an overworked musculoskeletal system. But real rest begins in the nervous system.

The secret to true, body-restoring rest is to allow the mind to relax — release it from a steady grind of work-thoughts or worries. Conscious thoughts take place in the Red. Red thoughts inspire Yellow override, and the Green responds with appropriate physiology. So the way your body is conducting business starts with conscious activity in your mind.

The mind and nervous systems need rest as much as the rest of the physical body. Sitting leisurely in a recliner may appear to relieve tension from a hard day's work, but when the mind goes full-tilt while the body relaxes, that's not resting.

Sleep allows for mind and body rest.

Yet many people wake as tired as they were when they went to sleep.

All too often problems of the day spill over to become problems of the night. And as far as confronting problems is concerned, the body has never learned to tell time. When the Red and Yellow "tell" the Green that trouble is afoot, the Green responds with defense. And defense means tension. So the body may be in a resting position, but both mind and body are tense. This tension can interfere with cell-replenishing, energy-restoring rest.

> WELLNESS PRINCIPLE: True rest comes when
> tension is released from
> both body and mind.

The thoughts and frustrations we take to bed with us often affect how we sleep and what we dream about. When your waking thoughts are concentrated on a particular problem or emotion, chances are that your "sleeping thoughts" will follow the same line.

Dreams might be considered to be animated thoughts. Often dreams are in full-color cinemascope. We might say that dreams are thoughts adapted for personal viewing. The word "dream" is defined as "Occurrence of ideas, emotions, and sensations during sleep."[79] It comes from an Anglo Saxon word meaning joy, glee, or happiness. But dreams can be far from joyful, gleeful, or happy. Nightmares are accompanied by fear. And fear, whether precipitated by dreams or life events, can affect your physiology while you sleep.

While nightmares may be sleep inspired fear, the emotions you take to bed with you can affect physiology and brain wave activity. Active beta waves at frequencies between 8 and 13 per second can be brought on by tension as well as intense mental activity. Slower theta waves, between 4 and 7 per second, occur during emotional stress, disappointment, and frustration in adults.

WELLNESS PRINCIPLE: Thoughts and emotions
                      affect the level of brain
                      activity.

When you go to sleep at night thinking about the problems and emotional upheavals of the day (or the past), these are the "sensory" signals your brain uses to determine the physiology appropriate for the moment. And since your brain doesn't understand the difference between internally generated stimuli originating from mental images and external stimuli originating from the five senses, it responds equally to both. But negative "sensory" emotions we take to bed with us are often intense. Here's where the Yellow comes in.

Intense emotions, along with their physiological responses, are recorded in Yellow. So when you go to sleep in the midst of intense emotions, the appropriate responses are "glued" in your Yellow. These memories of physiological responses can have a lasting effect on the way your body functions — and the way you

feel. That's why it is important that you put aside your worries
and frustrations before you crawl into bed and replace them with
strong positive feelings.

The Yellow "gluing" process works as well with positive
information as it does with negative information. Positive resting
thoughts adjust your physiology for restful sleep and calmer
wakefulness. Your Yellow is constantly at work communicating
with your Green, which directs physiology. So positive going-to-
sleep thoughts can be perpetual day-brighteners.

WELLNESS PRINCIPLE: Sleeping "glues" informa-
                       tion into your Yellow.

Since sleeping "glues" information into your Yellow, and
your Yellow provides constant "sensory" information to your
Green, what we need is an "exercise" that builds positive mental
response "muscles." And that "exercise" is *Forgiveness*.

CHAPTER 13

LEARNING EXERCISE

THE ULTIMATE EXERCISE

In an "ideal" world, there would be no disease, no physical pain, no mental pain, no anger, envy, anxiety, frustration, or other emotional upheaval. We would live free of crime, injustice, man's inhumanity to man, deception, and taxes. Our "ideal" world would be designed for our comfort. But we don't live in that sort of "ideal" world. Our world is not a haven of comfort. It isn't always user-friendly. So instead of our world being designed for us to enjoy care free living, ease, and pleasure, we are designed to survive in our less-than-ideal world.

We survive most comfortably when we understand that every experience we have in this less-than-ideal world is an opportunity for us to learn. And the biggest and most persistent lesson we must learn is that every experience contains within it a seed of "good."

Oh, I can hear the mental murmurs now: "He's quit preachin' and gone to meddlin'."

Meddlin' or not, my professional experience indicates that health — good or ill — springs from the mind and is manifest in the body. That's why we've been going on about Yellow override, memories of emotions, and all that. From my view of health, the Grand Designer didn't give us the ability to mess up

ourselves, our lives, and our health with negative emotional
memories without also giving us the ability to correct our mental
mistakes along the way. That's where forgiveness and "seeing
the good" in every situation come in.

> WELLNESS PRINCIPLE: Every experience is an
>   opportunity to affect your
>   health.

We have seen that Yellow override can keep the sympathetic
nervous system going full-tilt even though we think we are
resting and relaxed. Strong memories of Red perceptions with
intense emotions attached can keep the body ready to fight even
though the body appears to be relaxing.

If the Red conscious mind is behind the negative emotional
memories stuck in Yellow, the Red can be used to neutralize the
negative aspects of those memories. Red exercises of forgiving
and seeing the good can neutralize negative Yellow override.
Neutralizing Yellow override doesn't change the past or the
memories themselves. It removes, or lessens, the effect the
memories have on health. And it just might improve your
prospects for the future.

> WELLNESS PRINCIPLE: The seeds of Yellow over-
>   ride are planted by the Red.

Each of us has human reactions to our own life conditions.
And these reactions can keep us in a constant state of physiological defense. The purpose of the forgiveness exercise is to
improve your physiological responses. In the process, you will be
more relaxed both physically and mentally, and you will enjoy a
lot more.

You forgive for *your* sake — to improve your own condition.
When you are upset with someone, it's you who is affected, not
the other person. You can be very upset with your neighbor, but

your feelings don't keep the neighbor from going about his or her business and enjoying life. While you are fuming, nasty neighbor is still arranging a vacation to Hawaii or closing a lucrative business deal.

Perhaps the person you are upset with has died but you are still hanging on to your negative feelings about him. He probably wasn't affected by your strong negative emotions when he was alive, and he certainly isn't bothered by them now. So, if your negative thoughts and emotions have no effect on someone else — living or dead, your forgiving him won't affect him either.

> WELLNESS PRINCIPLE: You forgive others for *your*
>   sake, not theirs.

Forgiving an arch-enemy may appear on the surface to be noble and charitable, but the "forgiver" benefits more than the "forgivee." Now, that may sound selfish. But it's not. In order to help others, we must first have our own house in order. To be successful, your first priority is to keep yourself as mentally and physically healthy as possible. Your productivity, creativity, and service to family and community begin with you.

Forgiving isn't the same as excusing or approving of actions. We're talking about forgiving people, not actions. The forgiving doesn't change a situation, it changes your response to the situation. And since it's your responses that affect your physiology, you are the one who benefits from forgiving others. You don't have to like a person to forgive him or her. Your forgiveness won't change the other person in any way. But it may change your attitude toward him — even if the "him" is you.

Is all of this a take off on "forgive and forget"?

No, indeed.

We can't will ourselves to "forget" anything. The more we think about something, and the stronger we feel about it, the more firmly ingrained in memory it becomes. We don't forget incidents by forgiving the perpetrator. Forgiving tones down the physiological responses attached to strong emotional memories. That's why we need to forgive those who cause us grief.

WELLNESS PRINCIPLE: We need to forgive, because
we can't forget.

The idea of forgiving for health might seem simplistic and frivolous at first. We are accustomed to separating intangible emotions from the tangible physical. However, that tide is changing. We are coming to realize that thoughts, feelings, and emotions have a major influence on the physical body. Type A personality, stress, ulcers, hypertension, and all that. Actually, forgiving is a powerful process. It is neither simplistic nor frivolous. It can be fundamental to health, happiness, and success. Although the process of forgiving is simple, accomplishing the process may not be easy. However, establishing an exercise program of daily forgiveness can do more to improve your health than any other exercise you can do.

WELLNESS PRINCIPLE: Forgiving is one of the
most therapeutic exercises
you can give your body.

In the previous chapter, we talked about the "gluing in Yellow" factor of sleep. The strong thoughts, emotions, and accompanying physiological responses you take to sleep with you are glued into your Yellow. Once these emotions and responses are firmly nestled in Yellow, they can continue to provide Green with information. The validity of the Yellow based information is immaterial. The Green just keeps responding as though the actual situation that prompted the emotions is current. So, if emotions and responses are going to be glued into Yellow, it's just good common sense to make sure you neutralize the negative and "glue in" the most positive, physiologically neutral thoughts and emotions possible. That's what forgiving does.

WELLNESS PRINCIPLE: Forgiving generates positive, physiologically neutral
responses.

Bedtime is an ideal forgiveness time, but it's not the only time
for forgiving. When sincerely done, forgiveness works as well in
the middle of a turbulent day as it does before you go to sleep. In
fact, adopting a habit of forgiveness may take much of the
turbulence out of your days. And once it becomes a habit, it can
happen throughout the day automatically.

The forgiveness exercise takes some concentration. It is
simple, but you may find it hard work. And this concentrated
work is more easily accomplished when you are in the solitude
of your own thoughts. So, let's set the scene.

As you are tucked into bed ready for sleep, let your mind
follow its own path. If that path takes you on a journey through
the day's activities and tribulations, fine. If it takes you back in
time to past events, that's fine, too. Just let your thoughts go
where they wander.

As your mind wanders, it will probably stumble into the
memory of a disturbing situation — something that didn't go just
the way you would have liked it to go. The situation may have
occurred that day and is fresh on your mind, or it may have
happened long ago, or it may be something you think about often
that has no bearing on your activity at the time. The situation
may have involved one or more family members, co-workers,
business associates, friends, acquaintances, or strangers. Or it
may have involved only yourself.

Emotions that penetrate and become stuck in Yellow are
usually directed toward a person rather than toward an inanimate
object or condition. Let's suppose you are resentful at not having
enough money to live as comfortably as you would like. You
may be angry with the corporate wage policies where you work,

the government in general, or the IRS in particular for causing
your financial stress. However, corporations, the government,
and the IRS are nebulous groups of faceless people for most of
us. Nebulous groups don't make for effective forgiveness targets.
We need to aim our forgiveness energy toward a specific target.

So, whatever the situation, create a mental picture of an
individual. Your mental picture of this person may not be crisp
and clear, but a fuzzy mental picture of an individual is better
than a more clear picture of a building or large organization such
as the IRS. If the target of your budget-deficit ire is a boss, a
family member, or even yourself, that makes for easier visualiza-
tion. The main thing is to focus your thoughts on the person most
strongly involved. And, that person may be yourself.

First, we'll look at the steps of forgiveness, then we'll look
more closely at each step.

EXERCISING FORGIVENESS

Lie quietly with your eyes closed and create a mental picture of
the person involved. Think about the *feeling* attached to the
disturbing situation and the person. Once you are focused on the
feeling, go through the steps of forgiveness:

- Forgive the other person
- Forgive yourself
- Give the other person permission to forgive you

"What???" you ask incredulously. "I can go along with the
'forgive the other person' part. But, forgive myself and give that
so-and-so permission to forgive me? I'm the offended party!
Remember?"

Indeed. But before you conjure up another "forgivable
incident," remember that you are doing this exercise for your
sake, not theirs. You aren't putting your seal of approval on the
other person's actions. You are re-programming your Yellow
response to a past situation that can't be changed. And your
Yellow affects your life and health, not the other person's. So the
purpose is to improve your health and lot in life, not theirs.

WELLNESS PRINCIPLE: To forgive doesn't mean to
approve.

Step One: Forgive the Other Person
The first step of the forgiveness exercise is to forgive the other
person for whatever it was he or she did.

It is important to understand that the forgiveness exercise is
more than casual mental push-ups. Just thinking, "I forgive Uncle
George for abusing me when I was a child," doesn't get the job
done. The thought must be accompanied by sincere emotions of
forgiveness. None of this, "I forgive Uncle George — the jerk!"
When you forgive "Uncle George," be sure no strings are
attached. Even if Uncle George is no longer in the land of the
living, strong positive emotions of true forgiveness must
accompany the mental dialogue.

Forgiveness is an emotion — a feeling. *Actions are responses
to Red thoughts. Green-directed physiology is a response to
emotions.*

You may find it difficult to forgive "Uncle George" either
mentally or emotionally. His actions may have been reprehensi-
ble. However, they are in the past. Neither you nor he can do
anything to change things that have already occurred. But you
can change your attitude toward the memory of them. Physical
wounds from "Uncle George's" actions may have healed, but
continued anger and resentment can keep old emotional wounds
raw. And old emotional "wounds" that have never been allowed
to heal can lead to pain and ill-health.

In this first step, you begin to update Yellow patterns of
response to a painful memory of the past. Nothing about the
incident changes. But your attitude toward it begins to soften. In
the process, the defense physiology that the memory evoked is
reduced.

WELLNESS PRINCIPLE: Forgiving the other person
is an exercise in updating

emotions.

But suppose the person you are most upset with is yourself. What then?

The process is the same. You forgive yourself for your actions. You're not making excuses. You have already acknowledged to yourself that your actions were less than admirable, or you wouldn't be upset with yourself. An excuse is an attempt to rationalize in your Red thinking mind that what you did was alright. At a feeling level, you know it wasn't. Forgiveness is feeling. You acknowledge mentally and forgive emotionally.

When you are the center of this step of the forgiveness process, you are forgiving yourself for past actions just as you would forgive "Uncle George" for his actions. What's done is done. You can't change the past. So, for your health's sake, forgive yourself for your "sins of commission or omission." And learn from them. We all make mistakes. But the biggest mistake of all is to fail to learn from them.

> WELLNESS PRINCIPLE: An excuse is an act of
> conscious; forgiving is an
> act of conscience.

Step Two: Forgive Yourself
The second forgiveness step is to forgive yourself for any harm you may have done to yourself or to anyone else by your responses to the other person.

This is a very difficult step for many people, especially people who have a long-term specific physical complaint. When they realize that their anger, resentment, or other strong emotion connected with another person can be the underlying *cause* of their problem, they contract an instant case of the "guilts." Their first comment is something like: "You mean I did this to myself?" Now they have not only the strong left-over emotions from the incident, but strong fresh emotions of guilt.

Guilt is physiologically counterproductive. Guilt is self-directed. It affects the body just as much as any other strong emotion. And it's useless. We still can't change anything that's gone before. So there's no use feeling guilty about it. That's why this forgiveness step is so important. You don't need to get rid of one physiologically threatening emotion (anger, fear, frustration) and replace it with another (guilt). So, again, it's a process of acknowledging that your responses to the incident may have been responsible for doing yourself a physiological injury, and forgiving yourself for your actions.

Or, perhaps, your responses to the incident have had such an impact on your attitude and personality that you have made life miserable for your family and former friends who have dropped by the wayside. This step is where you forgive yourself — really forgive! with strong emotion! — for any harm you have done to others. The other people may never know about the forgiveness process you have gone through, but they will probably notice a difference in you.

WELLNESS PRINCIPLE: Forgiveness is an investment in your future.

Step Three: Give the Other Person Permission to Forgive You

The third step is to give the other person involved in the situation permission to forgive you for any harm you may have done to them.

"Hold on," you might think. "Now you're into blaming the victim."

No, indeed. Forgiveness isn't an exercise in assigning blame. It acknowledges that a wrong has been done, and it allows either the "wronger" or "wrongee" to accept responsibility for any part they played. Certainly, in some instances the "victim" is totally innocent. A child who is molested; the hapless and helpless victim of an intruder in the night; the unsuspecting occupants of a car struck head-on by an oncoming truck that crossed into their path. The world is full of innocent victims. Nevertheless, this step of the forgiveness process is important to innocent and guilty alike.

Most instances of "wrong" that breed health-debilitating emotions are less dramatic crisis events. They involve family, friends, and business associates. And in these relationships, rare is the conflict that is completely and absolutely one-sided.

Keep in mind that all of us are basically egocentric — "me-centered." Each of us views the world and the actions of others from our own personal perspective. We have our individual cocoon of attitudes, prejudices, values, and beliefs. From this perspective, all of our words and actions appear to be rational, logical, and true. Consequently, the other person may see the situation or incident that you find so distressing as logical and justifiable. It may have been just run-of-the-mill business or social intercourse. From that stance, your response of bitterness or anger appears wholly unjustified. The other person could probably assign you a degree of culpability, even if you are unaware of your role. You don't have to agree with the other person's assessment. However, for your forgiveness process to be effective, you do need to give him or her permission to forgive you in case you may have done something to offend them — even if you don't know what you're being forgiven for.

> WELLNESS PRINCIPLE: Allowing the other person
> to forgive you reinforces
> your forgiveness of them
> and yourself.

Forgiving is an exercise that directly benefits you alone. The feelings that come with sincere, industrial-strength forgiveness allow your body to release inappropriately-timed defense responses. In the process, organs, systems, and muscles that have been working overtime are allowed a little rest and relaxation.

Yellow override is reduced. Instead of your internal workings
responding to false alarm survival threats generated by your
Yellow, your body can limit its survival overdrive to responding
to external threats to physical survival. That's what your survival
systems were designed to do — protect you from oncoming
salivating tigers and club-wielding marauders.

You may be getting the idea that this forgiveness business is
heavy stuff. And it is. Understanding the power your emotions
and attitudes have over your life-circumstances can be a big step
in changing your life for the better. While forgiving can neutralize Yellow override and allow your physiology to shift out of
unnecessary high-intensity defense, to be even more effective,
there's more work to do. The objective is to learn how to change
your attitude toward negative experiences so that they become
positive learning experiences. Learning allows you to improve
your attitude and reduce the number of negative experiences that
need to be forgiven. That's the biggest challenge. But it's worth
the effort. And the way you learn from every negative lesson is
to find a seed of good in every experience.

> WELLNESS PRINCIPLE: Forgiveness is our way of
> dealing with the past; learn-
> ing the lesson is our way of
> preparing for the future.

A LIFETIME OF LESSONS
Picture a pre-toddler crawler who is working to gain his toddler
rank. (We will designate this imaginary toddler as a "he," and
name him "Chuck.") Chuck is a happy little fellow who has
watched the big people move about in an upright position. Looks
like fun. So, Chuck, being the little imitator he is, tries this
walking business himself. Although he is quite a clever small
person, he can't quite manage to raise up on his hind legs and
stride away all at once. He can pull himself up so that he is
looking at the world sideways instead of from the floor up. He

can take a few tentative steps, but he hasn't mastered the art of walking.

However, Chuck is not dismayed; he's learning. And one thing he has learned is that he hasn't mastered the refinement of moving in a straight line to get where he wants to go. He has a tendency to ricochet from obstruction to obstruction. He thumps a chair here, trips over a push toy there, clobbers his head on a low-slung coffee table, and tumbles off a step or two. Without conscious verbal analysis of these situations, Chuck is learning that there's more to walking than just putting one foot in front of the other. He learns from each "negative" walking experience how to do it better the next time. He learns not to try to stand up when he is under the coffee table, and to crawl down carefully from the precipices of stairs and chairs. Each "negative" walking experience gives him a chance to broaden his knowledge of how to get along in his world.

That's one of the things finding the seed of good does for us. It allows us to learn how to handle future obstacles. But more important, it allows us to replace feelings that can keep our physiology in fast-forward with feelings that are more user friendly.

When we forgive, we neutralize the effects of negative emotions. Finding the good in negative situations injects positive energy into the neutralized emotions. Forgiving handles situations of the past — finding the good prepares us for handling situations in the future. Forgiving by itself is about 40% effective. To be 100% effective, forgiving must be coupled with learning the lesson by finding and feeling the good.

> WELLNESS PRINCIPLE: Forgiving neutralizes long-term negative emotions; finding the good upgrades neutral to positive.

A response many of my patients have to the concept of feeling the good goes something like: "All well and good, but you don't understand the severity of what happened to me."

For example, one patient, at the age of about four or five, witnessed her father shoot and kill her mother. Although she was very young at the time, she remembered the scene vividly and could find absolutely no "good" in the situation. Yet she understood that her attitude toward her father and the situation in general was having a major effect on her health. After much work on extracting just a seed of positive from the experience, she realized that one positive aspect was that her father hadn't turned the gun on her. And, additionally, she realized that she had learned that she wanted to never inflict the kind of mental pain she suffered from the experience on anyone else. When she accepted that she had learned from her dreadful experience, she found that she felt more relaxed than she had in years, and her symptoms began to subside.

> WELLNESS PRINCIPLE: Until you learn the lesson, someone else is running your life.

Forgiving and finding the good may be the most strenuous exercise you can do. However, it might be more beneficial than physical exercise.

Physical exercise helps to improve muscle balance and tone, cardiorespiratory function, and internal communication. The emotional exercise of forgiving and learning the lesson allows the body to be in the physiological state most receptive to these improvements.

When your Yellow is filled with predominantly positive material, Yellow override is neutralized. And when Yellow override is neutralized, your body is relieved of the need to respond to outdated threats to survival.

> WELLNESS PRINCIPLE: Physiology should respond

to present, not past,
conditions.

When you understand and accept that health is a whole-body condition rather than merely a physical condition, you are on the way to living a more satisfying, productive, energetic life.

CHAPTER 14

FIELD EXERCISES

HEALTH RE-VIEW

How do you see your health and body? When you have an ache, pain, or illness that seems to crop up of its own volition, what do you see as the cause? Is it an organ or part that's run amuck? A system malfunction? A germ attack? Or, maybe, unbridled heredity? Those are the causes usually cited for physical distress that isn't prompted by an accident or other physical trauma. But, as I see it, those apparent causes are really effects. They are effects of the body following its natural instinct for survival. That's what we've been talking about in this book. How the body must adapt the way it functions to survive choices that cause undue stress. Symptoms, aches, and pains are signals that something is interfering with the designed functions of the body. And my experience indicates that interference affects the body's most basic communication system — energy.

One of the purposes of this book is to share with you my view of health as a whole-body condition. And that view includes more than the visible, tangible parts of the body. It includes the energy source that has been with each of us since we were one cell. From my perspective. . .

WELLNESS PRINCIPLE: The body is greater than the

sum of its parts.

Throughout this book we have been talking about how our body parts and systems respond. Internal systems don't make decisions or act independently. They respond to various stimuli. The stimuli are electrochemical in nature. So if organs and systems are responding in ways that result in discomfort, the place to look for the *cause* is at the lowest common denominator — the "power source" behind the stimuli that brought on the response. That lowest common denominator is subatomic energy.

WELLNESS PRINCIPLE: There's more to your body
                                    than meets the eye.

We live in a culture of components. Big things are made by putting together little things. Everything from towering skyscrapers to minuscule computer chips is a clever assemblage of bits and pieces. Small wonder, then, that we tend to think of our bodies as just another highly sophisticated assembly. And with life-saving procedures such as kidney dialysis, organ transplants, and heart by-pass surgery, our "culture of parts" is reinforced. This is good, especially if you or someone close to you gains additional years of life. But it isn't the whole story. There is a different way to look at health and the body.

As I see it, the most important area of health is energy transfer. From this perspective I see aches, pain, or illness as a snarl in the body's energy communication. Furthermore, I am now convinced that our choices in the six essentials affect our energy communication systems even before they affect the physiology of the visible physical body. That's what this chapter is about — my views and observations of the role of the energy of the body.

In chapter 6, we talked about energy — energy of mass and energy of motion. We also talked about and the unique, personal field of energy that is created when the fields of egg and sperm unite. It's that unique, personal field that controls development and function of the fertilized egg. Once the personal field is created, everything that happens in the body is a reflection of the vitality of that field.

Now, with this energy-inclusive view of the body, we'll look at how your body, life, and attitudes are affected.

THE BODY EXTENDED

We use energy and produce energy. And, at the most minute level, we are energy. My clinical experience indicates to me that the root cause of the physical complaints of my patients is interference in their complex energy network.

The energy network I'm talking about here is more than the energy that fires muscles and sends signals racing around nerve fibers. It's the "cloud" of "energy information" that surrounds every electron in the universe. The "energy information" of each electron is identical — each electron field has enough information to run the whole universe.

Electrons aren't isolated. They are everywhere all the time. They bump and collide and intermingle fields of energy information. Since we (and all other matter in the world) are made up of atoms with electrons and their fields, we are a part of that greater energy system. We function in and are part of *universal energy*.

> WELLNESS PRINCIPLE: We are not only *in* this
> universe, we are *of* the
> universe.

I envision the energy field of each individual as being like a personal "cocoon" around the body. We can't see this energy cocoon any more than we can see the force of gravity that keeps our feet firmly planted on earth, or the force of a magnet that grabs paper clips and other attractable metals. However, sensitive equipment can detect energy fields around the body. One example of this is Kirlian photography that produces "visual characteristics of an electrical corona."[80] As Dr. Robert Becker wrote in his book, *Cross Currents: The Promise of Electromedicine, The Perils of Electropollution*, "It may be a little disconcerting to know that we, and all other living things, are surrounded by a magnetic field extending out into space from our bodies, . . ."[81]

We might say that the surrounding energy field of a person is like that person's conjoined "identical twin." Everything that happens to one affects the other. As we shall see, the body can inject interference into the field which, in turn, interferes with transmission of information coming from the field. Body and field affect each other. And since your field is an extension of your body, the vitality of your field and the vitality of your body are equal. Strong, vibrant field — strong, vibrant body. Weak, puny field — weak, puny body.

Science has established the presence of fields. That isn't the issue here. The issue is, "So what?"

The big "So what?" is that we and our physiology work best when "energy information" flows freely between body and field. When the "flow" of energy between invisible field and physical body is hindered, both field and body are affected. Energy information between body and field flows best when body and field are "in tune" — that is, at the cellular level, the body "resonates" with the field at the same or compatible frequency. We call the results of synchronized rhythms of field and cells "health."

Energy "flow" is hindered when the rhythms of body and field are out of synch. Out of synch rhythms can produce less-than-desirable results. It's rather like having the woodwind section of a marching band playing and performing the routine for the school fight song while the rest of the band and the director are up to their crescendos in "Stars and Stripes Forever."

We might think of interference in energy flow as "noise" or "static" — extraneous signals that muddle transmission of information. The result of noise or static is a "power loss." Or to adapt a current heart disease metaphor, the "communication arteries" between field and body are so crammed with "plaque" that circulation of energy information is impaired. We can think of interference as "blocked information arteries" that result in a loss of power or energy.

> WELLNESS PRINCIPLE: Information blockage in the
>   field can bring on an
>   "energy attack."

As I see it, the energy field is perfect. If there is interference in transmission of energy between field and body, that interference originates in the body. Interference in communication between body and field impairs communication. And the primary source of interference is conscious thoughts.

ARE YOU INTERFERING?

The body is in the energy business — it is both producer and consumer. The body takes raw energy from the field and converts it to physiological energy. Activity in the brain uses and produces energy. Muscles rest occasionally, but the brain is continuously active.[82] The more activity in the brain, the more energy involved. The greater the excitement, the greater the intensity of brain activity.[83] And different centers of the brain react to particular qualities of information.[84]

> WELLNESS PRINCIPLE: Thinking is energy in
>   action.

For most of us, the most obvious "brain activity" is thinking — conscious thought. In order to think, the brain must be active. We usually think of the thinking part of brain activity as our "mind." Although "mind" is very difficult to define, for our purposes, we'll consider it the consolidated thinking or associative thinking activity of the brain — or as A.R. Luria put it, "a product of active processing of the flow of information working through elementary drives, or complex motives, set to single out important information about reality, . . ."[85]

We might say that thinking is a brain activity that influences and is influenced by the mind. It's as difficult to separate thinking activity from the mind as it is to separate the bat-swinging, ball-throwing, or running activity of baseball players from the baseball game itself. Inappropriate throwing, hitting, or running can interfere with the energy flow of a baseball game. And inappropriate thinking can interfere with the energy flow of the mind and field. Both thinking and playing baseball use and produce energy in a field setting.

Thinking and the mind are inseparable: thinking is a Red function, the "mind" is our connection with our field.

We said earlier that the energy field is the body's "identical twin" that controls the body. Thinking can affect the mind, and the mind can affect the field. Since the field controls the body, when the mind affects the field negatively, the results show up in the body. We call negativity in the field " interference."

WELLNESS PRINCIPLE: The field controls the body.

The way we think affects our fields. Positive thoughts allow uninterrupted energy communication between body and field. They are health-prone thoughts. Negative thoughts can interfere with body-field communication. If negative thinking is an occasional thing, the field effect is temporary. However, most of us think negatively most of the time. Interestingly, most of the patients who come to me believe they are positive thinkers. Yet after they analyze their thought process, most of the self-proclaimed positive thinkers realize that their thinking is habitually negative.

People believe what they think. They are positive that they are right. So they may think they are "positive thinkers" even when their thoughts are actually negative.

Negative thinking that affects your field and long-term health isn't the same thing as analyzing a situation and coming up with a negative response. Take the example of shopping for an insurance policy. After careful analysis of several policies, you reject policies "A" and "C" in favor of policy "B." That isn't negative thinking. That's practical, analytical thinking. Now, suppose that after you have done your analysis and made your selection, you find that an arch enemy from the past is now associated with company "B" and will profit from you buying that policy. Your rancor from years past is now injected into the analysis. Reasoned thinking gives way to negative feelings. These feelings become dominant. And we have seen that feelings run the body.

> WELLNESS PRINCIPLE: Negative feelings attached to thoughts can turn reasoning into negative thinking.

Negative thinking doesn't harm the body unless it is accompanied by strong, negative feelings. Physiology responds to feelings. One of our strongest negative feelings is fear. We have appropriate automatic physiological responses to fear that are designed to help us survive threats detected through our five senses. We learn what to be afraid of and to identify conditions that are perilous to our physical safety. This is the sort of information that is supposed to be stored in Yellow — information that will enhance our chances of survival.

However, along the path of growing up, we learn that life is full of threats that aren't a danger to the physical body. These threats are ego-bruisers, mental-zingers, and feelings-chafers — threats that are planted by the thinking Red mind and stored with feeling in Yellow memory where they are nurtured and sustained. As far as the body is concerned, memory or real, short-term or long-term, a threat is a threat, and the body responds with defense physiology. And the negative emotions can interfere with energy communication between body and field. Physiological responses to physical threats (such as the snake-stick) are usually short-term. The physiological and field repercussions from feelings attached to Yellow-stored threats can last for years.

> WELLNESS PRINCIPLE: Feelings are much more
> important than thoughts.

Negatives feelings such as anger, jealousy, guilt, resentment, anxiety, hatred, and the like, that are stored in Yellow not only keep your body inappropriately in defense, they project non-stop "noise" into your field. That's interference.

You may have noticed that we seem to have streaks of "bad luck." Often, when things begin to go wrong in life, problems begin as a trickle and grow steadily into a raging torrent. In the physical world, opposites attract. In the metaphysical world, likes attract. Negative feelings come in categories that attract experiences that produce similar negative feelings. Negatives put into the field attract similar negatives.

When difficulties are accompanied by negative feelings, that negativity makes its way into the field and attracts similar situations. This concept is often illustrated by those who careen from one crisis to another. They expect the worst from life, and they usually get it. From my perspective, these patterns are reflections of negativity that is introduced into the field.

> WELLNESS PRINCIPLE: Each of us is an expression
> of his or her personal field.

A full discourse on how I see the interrelationship of the field, mind, and body would fill several books. My purpose here is to offer my views, based on my clinical experience, of how thinking and choices in the six essentials can be major factors in health and success in life. Making better choices improves your chances of improving both your health and success. From this point of view, the very best way to improve your health is to direct your thinking so that your feelings inject the least amount of interference into your power field.

Am I saying that we can think our way into a smooth, carefree, crisis-free life?

Certainly not.

We have little control over many facets of our lives. However, we do have control over how — and how long — we respond to every situation. We know from experience that our responses to life circumstances affect our future. We are now coming to understand that our "mind" responses — thoughts, memories, and attitudes — affect our power source fields. With this understanding, these mind intangibles become main characters rather than "walk-ons" in our drama of life. Intangible thoughts, memories, and attitudes affect the condition of the personal field. The condition of the personal field determines the condition of the body. So thoughts, memories, and attitudes can be health-makers or health-breakers.

> WELLNESS PRINCIPLE: Your health is an expression
> of your field.

EXERCISE, ENERGY, AND THE FIELD

You might be wondering what your energy field has to do with exercise.

Exercise is important to your physical body and physiology. Exercise is one of the six essentials of life. However, your mental attitude toward exercise can affect your field. Most people are spurred to participate in exercise programs for one of three reasons: they enjoy the physical activity itself — it's fun; they anticipate enjoying the rewards of exercise — a slimmer, trimmer, better toned body and a more attractive appearance; or they are trying to improve their health — exercise is the "in" thing.

Exercise that is fun and stimulates the brain's pleasure centers as well as the metabolism is the most beneficial to the body as a whole. The pleasure may come from working toward reaching your personal best in weight-lifting, winning your club's tennis championship, or gliding as gracefully as possible around an ice skating rink. When you enjoy a particular type of exercise or sport, you and your muscles start out relaxed yet primed for action. Your body gets a good workout and you are less likely to suffer injuries. Exercise that includes contralateral movement gives you the added benefit of synchronizing your internal rhythms to resonate more closely with your field energy. In addition, you approach enjoyable exercise with a positive attitude. You don't fill your field with negatives when your attitude is positive.

> WELLNESS PRINCIPLE: Not thinking negatively is more important than thinking positively.

Exercising to lose weight, tone muscles, or generally improve personal appearance can have field-interfering elements.

Most people who enthusiastically launch an exercise program in an effort to slim down and shape up have a positive attitude at the outset. However, slimming, trimming results of exercise are rarely immediately apparent. Time and persistence are needed to reach body reshaping objectives. So the exercise program, the positive attitude, or both, tend to falter. Depending on the personality of the individual, the program is either abandoned or grudgingly continued. If it's continued, enthusiasm gives way to teeth-clenching tenacity. Positive feelings are replaced by negative feelings. Now the field is involved. The negative feelings can contaminate the field.

When exercising to reach a goal of losing ten pounds or sculpting abs, negative feelings related to the exercise can contaminate the field. Resentment and irritation toward the exercise can interfere with the energy of body and field. If the exercise you are doing stirs up negative feelings, you have two choices:

1.   Change your exercise routine to one that you enjoy, or

2.   Change your attitude so that you enjoy the exercise you have committed to.

WELLNESS PRINCIPLE: How you feel about the exercise you are doing affects
your field.

And then there are those who have been "alarmed" into exercising. This is the therapeutic, health-restoring approach to exercise. It may be prompted when a friend has a heart attack, or when the doctor tells them to do something to rouse their cardiovascular system to greater activity or suffer the consequences, or when an article on the perils of the sedentary life grabs their attention. Whatever the particulars of the motivation, health-restoration is the objective.

At the beginning of this book, we pointed out that exercise can't make you healthy. Certainly, exercise under duress is more beneficial to your heart and circulatory system than no exercise at all. However, when it comes to improving health, exercise is only one of the essential elements of your lifestyle. And when exercise is prompted by fear, the health-inhibiting effects of the fear may be greater than the health-enhancing effects of the exercise. Fear is a very strong feeling.

Feelings have a much greater effect on the field than thoughts. We can understand rationally that our bodies need exercise. However, emotional fear energy is stronger than rational thought energy. Which brings us to attitudes.

If your doctor tells you to exercise for your health's sake, follow his or her advice and be thankful. Your doctor is looking out for your physical welfare. It's up to you to look out for your attitudinal and emotional welfare. You can begin by focusing on the positive physiological benefits you get from the exercise. That's the find-the-good approach. Then choose to enjoy what you are doing. That reduces the amount of negativity that seeps into your field.

WELLNESS PRINCIPLE: Exercise a positive attitude.

CHAPTER 15

EXERCISING WITH ENERGY

EXERCISING BELIEFS

We have talked about the energy field that controls the body, and how the thinking mind can interfere with smooth communication between body and field. We can put those two principles together and see that the mind has a tremendous influence on the way the body works. Thoughts, memories, and attitudes can influence both life and physiology. We know that memories are based on our view of past experiences. But where do thoughts and attitudes come from?

They are based on our beliefs.

WELLNESS PRINCIPLE: Everything we think is colored by our beliefs.

We think the way we do because of our beliefs. Our thoughts, memories, and attitudes are products of our beliefs. And beliefs that stir strong emotions can affect health.

Beliefs, for the most part, come from interpretations of past experiences.

Our actions are colored by our beliefs. Politics, for example, are belief-based.

In politics, diverse beliefs are reflected as "liberal" and

"conservative" and debated as issues of the day. The results of political decisions may affect the quality of life. However, for the majority of people, political beliefs don't pack enough emotional energy to directly affect their health. On the other hand, religious and self-perception beliefs can be highly emotional. Those emotions can affect health.

> WELLNESS PRINCIPLE: Emotion-filled beliefs pack
> a physiological wallop.

Religion can be uplifting, inspiring, and hope-filled. Or, it can be oppressive, intimidating, and foster hopelessness and helplessness.

Religious beliefs that instill hope can be therapeutic. More and more doctors are beginning to acknowledge the power of prayer, or, if you prefer, "positive spiritual thoughts." However, some religious philosophies dwell on negatives and the inadequacies of the individual. These might be called "put down religions."

Now, I'm not trying to find fault with any religion. I am attempting to point out how beliefs, including religious beliefs, can affect health.

Some religious philosophies hold that anyone who doesn't believe or act in particular ways is doomed. If we really believe that the only way to a satisfying life or afterlife is to conform our thoughts and actions to a rigid set of guidelines, we set ourselves up for disappointment. Few of us can "religiously" conform to a precise set of standards without straying occasionally. Then, when we do miss the mark, we feel inadequate and guilty. Feelings of inadequacy and guilt are strong negatives. That's not to say that we shouldn't set high standards for ourselves and work to maintain them. We should. However, for our health's sake, we don't need to carry life-long guilt if we fall short once in a while. Mistakes in judgment are learning experiences. If we make the same mistakes over and over, we're not learning the lesson.

Religiously inspired guilt feelings are hard on the self-perception. More important, they are hard on the field. Our beliefs are with us constantly. Since we base our actions and thoughts on our beliefs, negative beliefs, such as "I am worthless" and "I am a sinner," transmit interfering energy to the field. And when there is interference in the field, there is interference in the body and life.

> WELLNESS PRINCIPLE: Religious beliefs can affect
> health, field, success, and
> satisfaction of life.

Philosophies and beliefs that foster negative feelings about oneself can have devastating physical consequences. We are very positive about our beliefs, and our actions reflect these beliefs. As mentioned earlier, nearly every patient who comes to me believes he or she thinks positively. And according to their belief systems, they are right.

Most of the people who come to my clinic are in major physical distress of some kind. Many of them have been to a variety of health care specialists and facilities looking for a "cure." According to their belief systems, doctors "cure" physical problems. And specialists "cure" specific physical problems. Yet, despite all of the doctors they have been to, they aren't "cured." When they get to my clinic, they not only have their physical problem but their long-held beliefs have been battered.

One of the first things I tell patients is that I don't "cure" anything. And I don't "treat" specific physical ailments. A body isn't made healthy by working on parts. The body is whole. When the whole body is healthy, the body itself will heal the parts.

My belief system about health is that the body doesn't "break down" by parts. Instead, interference in the body and field can reduce the efficiency of whole-body communication. This interference will show up first as symptoms in the "weakest link" of that individual. That "weakest link" may be revealed as physical symptoms relating to a part, such as the heart, pancreas, or skin. Or it might be manifest in the mental-physical symptoms we call depression. No matter which symptoms appear, my experience indicates that the ultimate cause is always the same — interference in the field. And the interference is generally belief based.

Having said all of that, how can you determine if your beliefs are undermining your health, happiness, and success? Check your current status.

> WELLNESS PRINCIPLE: Beliefs are expressed in the
> physical body and in
> patterns of life.

PERSONIFYING BELIEFS
We develop beliefs through experience and we live according to those beliefs — especially beliefs about ourselves. If we believe we are intelligent, attractive, successful, athletic, well-coordinated, generous, compassionate, or talented, we live and act accordingly. Or, if we believe we are none of the above, we still live and act according to our belief. It makes little difference whether or not our assessment is accurate. In the eye of the believer, the belief makes it true.

> WELLNESS PRINCIPLE: What you believe is what
> you get.

One clue that your beliefs may be undermining your life is that you are faced with the same type of situation over and over. A succession of similar negative experiences may indicate that false beliefs are driving actions. The results inject negativity into the field that attracts opportunities for repeat experiences. A succession of failed marriages. Lurching from job to job. Similar catastrophes or mini-catastrophes involving family or social relationships, finances, accidents, or health. It's the old "shoot yourself in the foot" phenomenon. It's such a common affliction that many self-help books have been written on the subject and described in a variety of ways — fear of success, the Cinderella principle, underachievment, or being motivationally challenged.

The most rampant negative belief among the patients I see is that of low self-esteem. Whether you see yourself as worthy of being all you can be or as being worth less than others colors how you respond to everything in your life. Your self-image is a picture that is the backdrop for every choice, decision, and direction your life takes. And your self-image has no bearing on your intelligence or any other characteristic.

> WELLNESS PRINCIPLE: Your self-worth and net-
>   worth are equal.

Self-image begins forming in childhood. Very few among us claim a perfect childhood. A child can develop a strong sense of helplessness and worthlessness from physical, psychological, or emotional mistreatment. Family members may or may not have been the culprits. The trauma could have been inflicted by schoolmates, neighbors, or friends. No matter the source, self-image forming incidents can range from simple verbal teasing to inhuman physical abuse. From the child's perspective, constant verbal put-downs can undermine self-esteem in much the same way as physical abuse.

> WELLNESS PRINCIPLE: We grow in maturity as we
>   grow in stature.

Our mental pictures of ourselves must be allowed to grow and change just as our physical stature grows and changes. If our beliefs fail to keep pace with the maturation process, we find ourselves hampered by outmoded beliefs as we try to function as adults. This is hardly a new concept. It is addressed in the Bible. "When I was a child, my speech, my outlook, and my thoughts were all childish. When I grew up, I had finished with childish things." (1 Cor: 13:11)[86]

Our beliefs are colored by our knowledge — or lack of knowledge. Only a few hundred years ago, even the best educated scholars believed that the earth was flat. Until recently, most of us held the general nutritional belief that we can't eat too much protein. And the belief that germs cause disease continues to flourish. As more and more is learned about our physical world and body, these and other generally accepted beliefs are falling by the wayside.

As this book is being written, we are hearing reports of the discovery of evidence of ice crystals on the moon. If confirmed, this is a belief-shattering discovery. Closer to home, archaeologists are finding evidence that indicates the historical accuracy of some biblical characters, including King David, whom many scholars consider to be mythical figures. So we can see that as knowledge expands, some of our beliefs are exploded and some are confirmed.

WELLNESS PRINCIPLE: Beliefs follow knowledge.

We readily adjust our beliefs to conform to new-found scientific and archeological evidence. Perhaps we need to reassess our beliefs about ourselves. Perhaps with a periodic reassessment of your beliefs about yourself you would find that your beliefs haven't kept up with your personal advances.

Your self-image is a powerful factor in your life. It governs how you respond to situations as minor as a surly comment by an overworked supermarket checkout clerk to career situations as major as applying for a better job. How you view yourself — your self-image, and how you feel about your worth as a person — your self-esteem, are among the strongest beliefs you hold. And since they are products of your mind, they can impact your health and field.

If your life isn't going the way you would like for it to go, you can inventory beliefs that could be obsolete or create static in your field. Identify beliefs that govern your actions and responses, and beliefs that lead you to respond the way you do to everyday situations. Your thoughts and beliefs should enhance your success, not stifle it. To help you begin to relate beliefs to actions, here are a few sample questions to get you going. Once you get the hang of it, you will come up with belief related questions of your own.

* Are juvenile beliefs conflicting with your adult life?
* Do you believe that your best efforts are never quite good enough?
* Do you find you are often treated with more respect or admiration than you believe you deserve?
* Are you surprised when your accomplishments outstrip your view of your ability?
* Do you believe you are destined to develop the same physical problems as your parents?
* Are you convinced that you must constantly be plagued by negative experiences of the past?
* Do you have the same types of negative thoughts day after day?

Your beliefs color your thoughts. Your thoughts influence your field and determine the way you respond to life. And the way you respond to every situation determines your health, happiness, and success. So take a hard look at the beliefs that guide your life. If you determine they are outdated, you can replace them the same way you formed them — by thoughts and feelings. Consciously changing your thoughts and feelings can help you update outdated or inaccurate beliefs.

We can ignore the impact the mind has on the body, health, and life and trust luck to solve problems that crop up in any of these areas. Or we can recognize the impact of the mind, work with it, and take control of our health, lives, and future. That's the forgiveness connection.

THE FORGIVENESS CONNECTION

There's no getting around it: life can be stressful. Many people seem to be afflicted with the "Scrooge syndrome." It's not that they are stingy and oppressive. Instead, they drag around a "heavy chain" forged link after link by major life stresses with only the occasional lighter link of benign tension. Each of today's stresses adds weight to their ever growing burden. A body becomes exhausted when it must continuously cope with the heavy chain of Yellow override stresses from the past on top of today's stresses.

That's where forgiveness comes in.

Forgiving and finding the good in every situation can update physiological responses to be more appropriate, and thereby help relieve residual physical tension. Now, when we add the field as a component of the communication system, forgiveness and finding the good takes on greater importance. Forgiving and finding the good can help reduce interference in communication between body and field. These two conscious activities are part of our learning process. There is no such thing as a negative lesson. Learning the lesson turns negative experiences into positive memories. And the biggest lesson we have to learn is that we are responsible for our own actions, thoughts, and feelings.

WELLNESS PRINCIPLE: Experiences are life's classrooms; forgiving and finding the good are the lessons.

Life is a learning process. "When you stop learning, you stop living" is more than a catchy saying. One of the biggest lessons we have to learn is that life experiences don't happen *to* us, they happen *for* us. Everything that goes on in your life is an opportunity for you to find an element of positive in that experience. That is why the forgiveness process we talked about in chapter 13 is so important. It helps you focus on positive elements in every situation. Negative thoughts reinforced with negative feelings contaminate your field. Positive thoughts, attitudes, and feelings are part of your personal anti-litter campaign — they reduce the amount of interference projected into your field.

If your attitudes and feelings are positive, they aren't negative. Feelings are more important than thoughts. Your Yellow is packed with every negative feeling you've ever had. Yellow-stored negative feelings can send inappropriate signals to your Green. And whether or not the signals from Yellow are appropriate, Green responses are always correct.

Yellow-stored negative feelings can "neutralize" energy from your field. Neutralizing acid in the body is good; neutralizing energy in the field isn't. So, instead of neutralizing the energy of the field, we would be much better off physically, mentally, and emotionally if we neutralize the effects of Yellow-stored feelings. And one way to do that is by applying the principles of forgiveness and, at the same time, involving the body's built-in survival mechanisms. Which brings us back to the forgiveness exercise with a twist.

As you go through the three steps of the forgiveness process — forgiving the other person, forgiving yourself, and giving the other person permission to forgive you — add the physical activity of holding your breath. That doesn't mean you should plop down on your bed, take a deep breath and hold it throughout the whole process. Each step gets its own separate breath-holding process.

Once you have generated a true feeling of forgiveness for the other person, close your eyes, think about that person with a positive feeling, take a deep breath and hold it as long as you can. Repeat the process for the next two steps — forgiving yourself and giving the other person permission to forgive you.

WELLNESS PRINCIPLE: For maximum   forgiveness
                      benefit, hold your breath.

Forgiving without holding your breath is a strong positive
force that can relieve tension and reduce defense physiology.
Forgiving — really forgiving — while holding your breath is the
most potent neutralizer of Yellow override that has been embedded by the experience (and person) being forgiven. It's based on
the principle of survival.

     Breathing is an ongoing essential. You can hold your breath
for only a matter of seconds or minutes. After that time, your
body is more interested in surviving the lack of oxygen than
anything else. At that point, lack of oxygen is a greater threat to
survival than the memory of the experience or person being
forgiven. Yellow override wastes energy. And since you are
focusing on the particular experience behind the Yellow override,
the brain is wasting a lot of energy on maintaining it. That
memory is "draining" energy. So the energy supply to that
particular memory is the first to be "shut down." In the process,
the strength of the negative aspect of the memory is reduced, or
neutralized. The memory itself is still there. But it is neutralized.
It is no longer a power-drain on the energy supply. In my clinical
practice, patients have told me that after "neutralizing" a
particular memory they not only think about the incident less but
when they do, the memory is less upsetting.

     We can't change the past. We can't undo things that have
been done, and we can't insert corrections into our past experiences. But we can neutralize the effects negative feelings toward
past experiences have on our future health and life.

WELLNESS PRINCIPLE: Your past is fixed; your cur-
                      rent responses to your past
                      are up to you.

EXERCISES IN THINKING

As functioning adults, we devote a lot of thought time to a variety of aspects of our person and personality — clothes, hair, cleanliness, appearance in general, social skills, career skills, diet, exercise, speech, and the countless other personal areas. But how often do we think about the way we think?

For many, thinking about thinking is a novel thought.

Yet we think every waking moment of our adult lives. And this important process affects every aspect of our lives. Why is it that we give so little thought to the process? Probably because thinking comes so naturally.

When we were children, our parents and teachers guided our information-absorbing thinking — or at least they tried to. As students, we recognized that what we thought about affected our school grades. As adults we recognize that what we think about affects our employment, income level, and relationships. But when it comes to thinking about what we think about when we're not thinking about something in particular, we rarely give it a thought.

For many people — especially the patients I see in my clinic — their thinking is punctuated by recurring mental re-runs of past negative experiences. It's not that they particularly want these thoughts to recur; the thoughts are just there. And as I examine these patients, I find that each time the patient thinks about the negative thought, his or her physiology and energy are affected — some area of the body becomes weaker.

> WELLNESS PRINCIPLE: Recurring negative thoughts
> waste energy.

Since most of us have a vast store of negative experiences packed away in our Yellows, most of us have recurring negative thoughts that promote muscle tension and drain our energy levels. One way to plug this energy drain is to identify the thoughts and neutralize them.

We can identify energy-draining recurring negative thoughts by noticing the first thing we think about when we wake up in the morning, or the last thing we think about before we go to sleep at night. One sign that recurring thoughts are more than just idle mental musings is that when they occur heart rate increases, breathing becomes deeper, or feelings of anxiety appear — Yellow override. If recurring thoughts alter physiology, you can bet that not only is your body responding to the thought, but your field is also responding. And your field is your connection with Universal Energy.

WELLNESS PRINCIPLE: Recurring negative thoughts
have far-reaching effects.

Once you have identified the thought or thoughts that are keeping your body stirred up and your field congested with static, what can you do?

Exercise forgiveness.

Neutralize communication-disturbing thoughts by going through the forgiveness exercise. We have seen that we can add power to the forgiveness process, by taking a deep breath and holding it. That works well as an end-of-the-day exercise. But you can also incorporate forgiveness into the Morter March. The physical exercise of the Morter March is vigorous but not strenuous. The mental exercise of forgiving may be strenuous, but it's not vigorous.

As you stretch through the Morter March, close your eyes, look up, take a deep breath, hold your breath and position, and think about the recurring thought that is interfering with your physiology and field. In this position, forgive the other person. When you must breathe again, relax for a moment. Follow this procedure for another Morter March step and forgive yourself. Then finish the exercise with another Morter March step and give the other person permission to forgive you.

The Morter March by itself helps to re-time muscles and

internal communication systems. The Morter March combined with holding your breath and forgiving or focusing on a particular area of Yellow override coordinates the mental and emotional with the physical. Whole-body communication is improved. Since your field is an integral part of your body, this exercise is a comprehensive whole-body exercise.

WELLNESS PRINCIPLE: Strong thoughts and retiming action incorporated with positive feelings re-energize mind, body, and field.

Exercise is one of the essentials for whole-body health. Your body needs exercise. It needs exercise to keep it in the best shape possible for survival. Our caveman ancestors didn't need to schedule exercise time. If they weren't strong and didn't move well, they didn't survive. But life is a lot easier now. We forage for food in a supermarket instead of the wild, and we wheel from place to place instead of walking or running. So, now, we must make a conscious effort to exercise muscle and sinew.

Exercise is one of the six essentials. Contralateral exercise, such as the Morter March, can help retime the body's internal communication systems, improve muscle tone, and boost cardiovascular efficiency. But the best health-enhancing exercise is exercising discretion in all of the six essentials — eating, drinking, resting, breathing, exercise, and thinking.

And that's what this book is all about.

The underlying theme of this book is that everything that happens in and to any part of the body affects the whole body — including the body's energy field. What we eat and drink, how we rest, breathe, and exercise, and what we think either enhances or diminishes the health of the whole body. All of the six essentials are important. Although we have been led to believe that diet and exercise are the principal determinants of health, in reality, thoughts are at the top of the importance scale.

WELLNESS PRINCIPLE:　Just eating right and
exercising won't guarantee
health.

Each of us is responsible for his or her own health. And each
of us has the opportunity to improve his or her own health. We
increase the likelihood of good health when we allow the body to
function at its best most of the time. That means following a
well-rounded routine of making the best choices possible in the
six essentials.

To summarize the guidelines for making better choices in the
six essentials:
- Eat more fruits, vegetables, and whole grains, and less meat,
poultry, and fish.
- Drink pure, chemical-free water when you are thirsty. With a
diet that includes a lot of fruits and vegetables, you won't be
as thirsty as you will with a diet that is meat-centered.
- Rest as much as your body dictates. Avoid sleeping pills and
alarm clocks.
- Breathe fresh air as much as possible. If you can smell man-
made aromas, the air you are breathing may be harmful to
your health.
- Exercise regularly with contralateral movement. Slow
walking helps reestablish metabolic balance. Include the
Morter March to promote a full range of motion.
- And, most important, think about what you think about.
Recognize negative thoughts. Find a seed of positive in the
experience and replace the negative thought with a positive
thought and positive feeling.

Keep in mind that your body is designed to heal itself. And it
does that very well when interference is kept to a minimum. The
choices you make in the six essentials determine the amount of
interference your body must contend with. When you make

correct choices, you allow your body the opportunity to do its job in a way that leads to health, happiness, and success.

      WELLNESS PRINCIPLE: Health, happiness, and success are inside jobs.

ENDNOTES

1. *Taber's Cyclopedic Medical Dictionary*, 15th Edition,
    Thomas, Clayton L., Editor. Philadelphia: F.A. Davis
    Company, 1985.

2. Guyton, Arthur C., M.D. *Human Physiology and
    Mechanisms of Disease*, 3rd Ed. Philadelphia: W.B.
    Saunders Co., 1982, p. 37.

3. Ibid, p. 265.

4. Guyton, Arthur C., M.D. *Textbook of Medical Physiology*,
    7th Edition. Philadelphia: W.B. Saunders Co., 1986, p.
    382.

5. Bailey, Covert. *Smart Exercise: Burning Fat, Getting Fit*.
    Boston: Houghton Mifflin Co., 1994, p. 225.

6. Guyton. *Textbook of Medical Physiology*, 7th edition, p.
    643.

7. Ibid., p. 133.

8. Ibid., p. 608.

9. Stamford, Bryant A., PhD. *Fitness Without Exercise: The
    scientifically proven strategy for achieving maximum
    health with minimum effort*. New York: Warner Books,

Inc., 1990, p 80.

10. Mountcastle, V. B., Ed. *Medical Physiology*, 12th edition, Vol. II. St. Louis: The C.V. Mosby Co., 1968, p. 1128.

11. Guyton, *Textbook of Medical Physiology*, p. 130.

12. Ibid., p. 134.

13. Ibid., p. 1013.

14. Ibid., p. 134.

15. *Taber's Cyclopedic Medical Dictionary*, p. 520.

16. Ferris, Timothy, Editor: *The World Treasury of Physics, Astronomy, and Mathematics*. Boston: Little, Brown and Co., 1991, p. 26.

17. Ibid., "Atoms in Motion," Richard P. Feynman, p. 8.

18. Guyton, *Human Physiology and Mechanisms of Disease*, 3rd edition, pp. 548-9.

19. Ibid.

20. Ibid., p. 549.

21. Ibid., pp. 530-1.

22. Klivington, Kenneth. *The Science of Mind*. Cambridge, MA: The MIT Press, 1989, p. 155.

23. Guyton, *Human Physiology and Mechanisms of Disease*, 3rd edition, p. 84.

24. Chopra, Deepak. *Quantum Healing: Exploring the Frontiers of Mind/Body Medicine*. New York: Bantam Books, 1989, p. 48.

25. Magoun, H.I., Sr. *Osteopathy in the Cranial Field*, Third ed. Kirskville, MO: Journal Printing Co., 1976, pp 23-4.

26. Guyton, *Human Physiology and Mechanisms of Disease*, 3rd edition, p. 28.

27. Chopra, *Quantum Healing: Exploring the Frontiers of Mind/Body Medicine*, p. 45.

28. Guyton. *Human Physiology and Mechanisms of Disease*, 3rd edition, p. 571.

29. Ibid, pp. 571, 590.

30. Tuttle, W.W. and Byron A. Schottelius. *Textbook of Physiology*, 14th edition. St. Louis: The C.V. Mosby Company, 1961, p. 377.

31. Guyton. *Textbook of Medical Physiology*, 7th edition, p. 692.

32. Guyton. *Human Physiology and Mechanisms of Disease*, 3rd edition, p. 444.

33. Guyton. *Textbook of Medical Physiology*, 7th edition, p. 692.

34. *Health*, Mar/Apr 1994, Vol. 8, No. 2, p. 70.

35. *Health*, Mar/Apr 1994, Vol. 8, No. 2. p. 70.

36. Fiatarone, Maria A., M.D., Director. *Get Ready to Exercise*. Boston, MA: Fit for Your Life, 1992, p. 4.

37. White, Timothy P., PhD. *The Wellness Guide to Lifelong Fitness*. New York: Random House, 1993, p. 10.

38. Tuttle and Schottelius, p. 326.

39. Guyton. *Textbook of Medical Physiology*, 3rd edition, p. 942.

40. Ibid, p. 943.

41. Ibid.

42. Tuttle and Schottelius, p. 330.

43. *Health*, May/June 1996, Vol 10, No. 3, p. 131.

44. Shute, Nancy. "Get Fit in a Flash," *Health*, Jul/Aug 1996, Vol. 10, No. 4, p. 40.

45. Poppy, John. "Walk This Way," *Men's Health*, Oct 1994, p. 118.

46. Guyton, *Textbook of Medical Physiology*, 7th edition, p. 610.

47. Sun, Wei Yue, M.D. & Chen, William, Ph.D., *Tai Chi Ch'uan: The gentle workout for mind & body*. New York: Sterling Publishing Co., Inc. 1995, pp 6-13.

48. Bailey, p. 103.

49. *Taber's Cyclopedic Medical Dictionary*, 15th edition, p. 1126.

50. Guyton. *Textbook of Medical Physiology*, 7th edition, p. 506.

51. Tuttle & Schottelius, 14th edition, p. 390.

52. Guyton. *Textbook of Medical Physiology*, 7th edition, pp. 506-7.

53. Ibid, p. 502.

54. Mountcastle, Vol. I, p. 473.

55. Ibid, p. 473.

56. Guyton. *Textbook of Medical Physiology*, 7th edition, p. 808.

57. Ibid, p. 809.

58. Ibid, p. 808.

59. Ibid, p. 809.

60. *Taber's Cyclopedic Medical Dictionary*, 15th edition, p. 691.

61. Ibid, p. 1037.

62. Guyton. *Textbook of Medical Physiology*, 7th edition, p. 813.

63. *Taber's Cyclopedic Medical Dictionary*, 15th edition, p. 691.

64. Guyton. *Textbook of Medical Physiology*, 7th edition, p. 810.

65. Ibid, p. 816.

66. Ibid, p. 813.

67. *Taber's Cyclopedic Medical Dictionary*, 15th edition, p. 44.

68. Ibid, p. 921.

69. Guyton. *Textbook of Medical Physiology*, 7th edition, p. 1010.

70. Ibid, p. 1011.

71. "Berkeley Wellness Letter," Vol. 12, Issue 10, July 1996, p. 6.

72. Ibid.

73. Ibid.

74. *Taber's Cyclopedic Medical Dictionary*, 15th edition, p. 1573.

75. Ibid, p. 853.

76. Carey, Benedict. "The Slumber Solution," *Health*, July/Aug 1996, Vol. 10, No. 4, p. 72.

77. Ibid.

78. Bailey, p. 97.

79. *Taber's Cyclopedic Medical Dictionary*, 15th edition, p. 491.

80. Gerber, Richard. *Vibrational Medicine: New Choices for Healing Ourselves*. Sante Fe, NM: Bear & Company, 1988, p. 53.

81. Becker, R.O. *Cross Currents: The Promise of Electromedicine, The Perils of Electropollution*. Los Angeles: Jeremy P. Tarcher, Inc., 1990, p. 70.

82. Guyton. *Textbook of Medical Physiology*, 7th edition, p. 669.

83. Ibid.

84. Ibid, p. 661.

85. *The Oxford Companion to the Mind*, Gregory, Richard L., editor. New York: Oxford University Press, 1987, p 489.

86. *The New English Bible*: *The New Testament, Oxford Study Edition*. New York: Oxford University Press, 1976. p. 213.

INDEX

fruit 29-34, 101
gastric 42
germs 145, 231
grains 25, 27, 29, 33, 91, 239
guilt 15, 45, 47, 59, 107, 140,
   208, 221, 227, 228
heredity 80, 214
homeostasis 2, 42, 54, 116,
   127, 195
hypothalamus 40, 41, 58
indecision 40
interference 99, 100, 103,
   142, 184, 185, 214,
   216-219, 221, 222,
   228, 229, 233, 234,
   239, 240
judgment 227
kidneys 19, 26
lesson 52, 64, 65, 73, 115,
   117, 200, 210-212,
   228, 233
memories 34, 45, 47-52, 55,
   59, 62, 70, 100, 117,
   144, 145, 160, 188,
   195, 198, 200, 201,
   203, 222, 226, 233
memory 37, 49-51, 54-57, 59,
   69, 70, 109, 117, 118,
   144, 186, 202, 204,
   206, 220, 235
milk 31, 33, 34, 178
minerals 28-30, 32, 34, 73,
   92, 167
Morter March 153-161, 165,
   167, 185, 237-239

neutralize 27-29, 32, 51, 52,
   145, 161, 169, 201,
   203, 210, 211,
   234-237
nutritional stress 103
oxygen 4, 7, 12, 13, 17, 27,
   31, 40, 75, 81, 89-92,
   106, 120, 126, 127,
   132, 147, 148, 158,
   159, 165, 168, 171,
   172, 174-179,
   181-183, 185, 235
pain 1, 8, 9, 11, 15, 17, 19,
   22, 48, 59, 61, 62,
   64-66, 74, 109,
   117-120, 125, 130,
   137, 154, 164, 188,
   192, 194, 195, 200,
   206, 212, 214, 215
parasympathetic 42, 43, 76,
   112, 114-117, 148,
   195
perfect 12, 16-18, 33, 57-61,
   99-102, 114, 119, 131,
   143, 144, 159, 163,
   192, 218, 230
perfection 59, 118
pH 152, 173, 180
pollution 32, 169, 170
priority 30, 182, 202
protein 24, 25, 27, 28, 73,
   111, 123, 134, 167,
   172, 180, 181, 231
proteins 174
pulse 195